FAME JUNKIES

Books by Jake Halpern

Braving Home

Fame Junkies

.

Jake Halpern

F★AME
junkies

The Hidden Truths Behind
America's Favorite Addiction

Houghton Mifflin Company
2007 • BOSTON • NEW YORK

Library of Congress Cataloging-in-Publication Data
Halpern, Jake.
    Fame junkies : the hidden truths behind America's favorite
addiction / Jake Halpern.
            p. cm.
    Includes bibliographical references.
    ISBN-13: 978-0-618-45369-6
    ISBN-10: 0-618-45369-5
    1. Subculture—United States. 2. Fans (Persons)—United
States—Psychology. 3. Fame—Psychological aspects. 4. Celebrities
—United States. I. Title.
    HM646.H35   2007
    306.4'87—dc22   2006011143

Book design by Melissa Lotfy

PRINTED IN THE UNITED STATES OF AMERICA

MP 10 9 8 7 6 5 4 3 2 1

To my brother, Greg

Rather than love, than money, than fame, give me truth.

—HENRY DAVID THOREAU, *Walden* (1854)

Contents

Introduction: Hooked on Fame

Several months before he became famous, seventeen-year-old Jerrell Jones visited the Black Pearl tattoo parlor, in downtown St. Louis, and made an unusual request: he wanted a six-inch-long bar code, complete with a minute serial number, etched on his forearm in dark-green ink. As far as Jones was concerned, his decision to get the tattoo was just one more step on the path to fame. Prior to this, he had run away from his home in the suburbs and spent several months living the life of a vagabond on the streets of St. Louis, sleeping in abandoned cars and writing rap lyrics by the flame of a cigarette lighter. During this time he renamed himself J-Kwon, and began to prepare for the fame he felt was imminent. "I got the bar code because I knew that someday I'd be a product," he told me in 2003. "I knew they were going to sell me."

He was right.

J-Kwon eventually enlisted the help of two local rap producers, known as the Trackboyz. Together they recorded his debut album, *Hood Hop,* and sold it to Arista Records. It wasn't long before hangers-on began to swirl around J-Kwon like debris in a cyclone. They included several personal assistants, one of whom was a teenager known as "Versatile"—though J-Kwon soon renamed him "Four," in homage to the rapper Nelly, who apparently had an assistant named "Three." Another member of J-Kwon's extended entourage was an almost-famous rapper named 40 Grand—or "Uncle 40," as J-Kwon sometimes called him—whose primary job was to recount his own failures and serve as a kind of living cautionary tale. The dozen or so members of J-Kwon's entourage followed him around, gave him advice, offered him protection, lavished praise on him, and did whatever they could to seal their mutual fate and garner a one-way ticket out of obscurity.

As J-Kwon's hit song "Tipsy" began to get more airplay, the frenzy surrounding him mounted. While visiting a Foot Locker at a St. Louis shopping mall, he drew such a crowd that mall officials closed off the store and asked him to call ahead in the future so that they could arrange for extra security. After a show in Birmingham, Alabama, a mob of fans grew so rowdy that J-Kwon needed a police escort back to his hotel. In Los Angeles, which he visited to appear on *The Tonight Show with Jay Leno,* a woman approached him and said that the seventeen-year-old rapper had changed her life and that she wanted to have his baby.

In the span of just a few months I witnessed J-Kwon evolve from a marginalized teenager into a bona fide celebrity. I chronicled much of what I saw in an article for *The New Yorker,* but long after its publication the story remained firmly embedded in my thoughts. Talk of celebrities may be ubiquitous, but fame itself is still the rarest of commodities. And everybody—including J-Kwon, Uncle 40, Four, the screaming hordes in Alabama, the would-be mother to his child in Los Angeles, and me—all of us were beguiled by it. On some fundamental, almost primal level, it seemed as if we were all hungry for a taste of it.

I will be the first to admit that writing about fame is a stretch for me. I grew up far from the glitz of Hollywood, in the Rust Belt city of Buffalo, New York, with a leftist father who for years wore a massive Castro beard, and a mother who accumulated advanced degrees but, despite my best efforts to teach her otherwise, constantly confused Bob Marley with Barry Manilow. The closest I got to "glamour" was donning my moon boots and polar parka to trudge through the snow for a screening of *Wres-*

tleMania at my neighbor's house. Even years later, during my first encounter with a Hollywood agent, I asked so many obvious and apparently naive questions that he finally snapped, "Kid, where the hell are you from, Buffalo?"

My first real exposure to celebrity culture was in the mid-1980s, during my early adolescence, when my parents briefly acquiesced to my demands for cable television. Almost immediately my show of choice became *Lifestyles of the Rich and Famous,* which first aired in 1984. On wintry evenings, as gale-force winds howled through the deserted streets of North Buffalo, I cozied up to the warm glow of the TV and let the host, Robin Leach, whisk me into a rarefied world of private yachts and gold-plated bathroom fixtures. Perhaps needless to say, these things weren't too common in Buffalo—especially during the 1980s, when the city was still reeling from the loss of the steel industry.

Looking back, it seems odd to me that *Lifestyles of the Rich and Famous* was so popular. In other times and places the flaunting of such discrepancies in wealth has incited revolution, but for some reason this show did precisely the opposite: it enthralled millions of middle-class viewers like me. I was a ridiculously skinny, uncoordinated kid, so I avoided sports, read way too many books, and talked pretty much continually. I must have set off an almost Pavlovian response in schoolyard bullies. Robin Leach seemed to provide a reprieve from all this. For thirty minutes his show allowed me to escape from the cramped confines of our family room—with its water-stained ceiling and buzzing radiators—and enjoy an intoxicating dose of glamour.

One of the many things that still fascinate me about *Lifestyles of the Rich and Famous* is that no rich or famous people were actually on the show. We, the viewers, saw only these people's possessions. In a way, the whole show functioned as one continuous "point-of-view shot," which is what facilitated the voyeurism of it all. And I'm pretty sure that's why I liked the show so much. Once a week it allowed me to imagine that I was in Malibu, or Beverly Hills, mingling with the glitterati, barking orders at my butler, or receiving fan mail in my mahogany-paneled study. At the time, I was only nine years old, but I was clearly already nursing delusions of grandeur and beginning to fixate on the idealized notion of what it meant to be a celebrity.

My parents eventually became so annoyed with my weekly devotion to *Lifestyles of the Rich and Famous* that they actually gave away our television set, thus ending my obsession with Robin Leach and the world he advertised. To fill the void they bought me a bicycle, and when the weather permitted, I channeled my time and energy into cycling. Still, I suffered momentary relapses. I'd go to a friend's house for a sleepover, and before I knew it I was glancing at the television and pining for the sound of Robin Leach's English accent.

Even today a similar urge lingers. The big difference now is the number of "celebrity news" outlets. All you have to do is click on E!, the twenty-four-hour celebrity-news network, or buy a copy of *Us Weekly* and turn to the "Stars—They're Just Like Us!" section for news about Brad and Angelina's latest tropical vacation. And I still get sucked in. I'll be walking through an airport, hustling toward my gate, and the next thing I know I'm standing beneath a television set, watching a segment on Julia Roberts's adorable children. As I'm absorbing every last word of this pap, somewhere in the back of my head the faintest of voices is asking, "Why on earth do you care?"

Joel Resnick is a red-carpet dealer. On any given day he has about 3,000 yards of red carpet at his office in Flemington, New Jersey. He runs the Red Carpet Store, one of the nation's leading suppliers of special-event carpeting. His company's Web site notes, "Whether you are looking for a way to elevate your private party to a 'Red Carpet' event, are catering to the Stars, or are looking for a conversation piece for your own home, the Red Carpet Store has got you covered." Resnick has been in the red-carpet business for only a few years, but he has already made quite a name for himself: he did the carpeting for the MTV Music Awards and the 2004 Summer Olympics, among other events.

Resnick does much of the work himself—he takes the orders, cuts the materials, binds the edges, and ships the carpets. Sometimes, when the event is in New York City, he actually nails the carpet to the floor on-site. He first did this for the 2003 MTV Music Awards, and what he saw there made a huge impression on him. As he was laying the carpet, die-hard fans begged him for scraps. Not wanting to disappoint them, Resnick tossed over a few frayed strips of red cloth and watched in amazement as the fans gushed with appreciation. Afterward he began selling larger (two-foot-square) souvenir swatches on eBay for $20.00 apiece.

"Selling red carpets is a high profit margin," Resnick told me. "It is relatively cheap material and people are willing to pay top dollar for it, and that is a beautiful thing." When I asked him why Americans are so captivated by red carpet, he was quick to answer: "It's like diamonds. They are not actually that rare, but the minute kings and queens started wearing them, everyone wanted them." It's all about the power of association, concluded Resnick, and in this instance our obsession with celebrities has simply carried over into the realm of fabrics.

Resnick's story isn't all that surprising. After all, we live in a country where the ultimate competition for celebrityhood—*American Idol*—has more viewers than the nightly news on the three major networks combined. And our interest in celebrities doesn't appear to be waning. The circulation of the major news and opinion magazines (including *Time, Newsweek, The New Yorker,* and the *Atlantic*) increased by only 2 percent between 2000 and 2005, while the circulation of the major entertainment and celebrity news magazines (including *People, Us Weekly, InStyle,* and *Entertainment Weekly*) increased by 18.7 percent. The cult of celebrity is also making an impact on the $175 billion clothing industry. In 2002 celebrity labels accounted for just 6 percent of this industry; by 2005 that number had jumped to more than 10 percent. Industry analysts expect it will hit 15 percent by 2009. But perhaps the most telling statistics involve our heroes. Ever since the early 1960s the Gallup Organization has been conducting a poll about which man Americans most admire, and compiling a list of the top twenty or so overall finishers. In 1963 that list included a number of political figures—Lyndon Johnson, Winston Churchill, Charles de Gaulle, and Martin Luther King Jr. among them—but not one entertainment celebrity, sports star, or media personality. By 2005 the list included six such people: Mel Gibson, Donald Trump, Bono, Michael Jordan, Arnold Schwarzenegger, and Rush Limbaugh.

More worrisome than any of this, however, is the effect that our national obsession with fame and celebrities has on children—especially girls. A survey I organized, with the generous help and guidance of statisticians at Boston College and Babson College, yielded some interesting findings. The survey was distributed to 653 middle school students around Rochester, New York, a community whose demographics in many ways reflect those of the nation as a whole. In one question students were asked to choose from a list of famous people the one they would most like to have dinner with. There were a range of options including "None of the above." Among the girls who opted for the dinner, the least popular candidates were President George W. Bush (2.7 percent) and Albert Einstein (3.7 percent). Far ahead of them were Paris Hilton and 50 Cent (15.8 percent each), who tied for third place. Second place went to Jesus Christ (16.8 percent), and the winner was Jennifer Lopez (17.4 percent). Another question asked, "When you grow up, which of the following jobs would you most like to have?" There were five options to choose from, and among girls, 9.5 percent chose "the chief of a major company like General Motors," 9.8 percent chose "a Navy Seal," 13.6 percent chose "a United States Senator," 23.7 percent chose "the president of a great university like Harvard or Yale," and 43.4 percent chose "the personal assistant to a very famous singer or movie star."

It is commonly said that Americans are obsessed with celebrities, but this observation raises the question, What, exactly, makes someone a celebrity? Indeed, the word "celebrity" seems to encompass everyone from high-profile sushi chefs to Olympic shot-putters to Supreme Court justices. But for the purposes of this book I was most interested in the quintessential entertainment celebrities—J-Kwon, Brad Pitt, Madonna, even Paris Hilton—whom we often see parading down the red carpet. I wanted to know, Why do countless Americans yearn so desperately for this sort of fame? Why do others, such as celebrity personal assistants, devote their entire lives to serving these people? And why do millions of others fall into the mindless habit of watching them from afar?

In search of answers, I began to imagine a journey of sorts—a plunge into the vortex of fame, where celebrity was not just a persistent distraction but a full-blown, all-encompassing obsession. My plan was to examine three separate subcultures: the first inhabited by aspiring celebrities, the second by personal assistants and other entourage insiders, and the third by die-hard fans. Each subculture is the focus of one section of this book.

Before I went anywhere, however, I wanted to consider some of the ideological underpinnings of fame. Admittedly, I'm not the first to grapple with this issue: over the course of history, everyone from Virgil to Kitty Kelly has taken a stab at understanding the workings of fame. And this is as it should be, for the story of fame is an ancient one.

Many cultural anthropologists believe that even the hunters and gatherers of the Stone Age—who are thought to have lived in a relatively egalitarian fashion—had top hunters who enjoyed a special celebrity-like status. Kristen Hawkes, of the University of Utah, has spent years studying the Hadza, an isolated tribe of roughly a thousand hunters and gatherers who live near Lake Eyasi, in northern Tanzania. According to Hawkes, the best Hadza hunters typically have the privilege of marrying the women who are most adept at gathering, and often they use their status to marry young and fertile second wives. The boys in the tribe follow the exploits of these hunters with great zeal. "It's almost like these boys are following the statistics of their favorite sports stars," Hawkes told me. All of this supports her theory that the best hunters are essentially obsessed with their reputations and with showing off for the other members of the tribe. "Hadza hunters generally pass up chances to hunt and kill small animals that would be a welcome addition to their families' cooking pots," she explained. "Instead they go after the big animals—the giraffes, the buffalos, and the zebras—which carry enough meat to feed several villages and which, when killed, generate great stories and tremendous buzz." What makes the Hadza tribe so interesting, insists Hawkes, is that they live in a place where people have been hunting and gathering in the wild for almost two million years. Indeed, the stone tools and the bones of large mammals that archaeologists have found in the nearby Olduvai Gorge serve as our oldest evidence of how ancient humans lived. So the grandstanding Hadza hunters of today may offer a glimpse into the distant past, when early man vied mightily not just for survival or power but also for reputation and fame.

Of course, the notion of celebrity in the modern sense of the word didn't really take hold until the Industrial Revolution, with the advent of the telegraph, the telephone, and eventually the radio—technologies that greatly expedited the process of becoming famous. Previously, stories about Genghis Khan or Alexander the Great had taken hundreds if not thousands of years to saturate the public consciousness, whereas suddenly someone's story could spread widely within a matter of weeks, days, or even minutes.

One could argue that all the celebrity hoopla we see today is simply the inevitable result of technology, which now disseminates countless images and stories in nanoseconds. But theoretically this same technology also makes it infinitely easier to spread scientific knowledge or historical records. So why have we not become a nation of obsessive science geeks or fanatical history buffs? The answer may be that technology has simply made it much easier for us to act on impulses that have been with us since the beginning—namely, the impulses to admire others and to be admired ourselves. The question then becomes, Has technology amplified these impulses, not just around the world but within each of us as well? In other words, to what extent can we blame *Lifestyles of the Rich and Famous* or *Entertainment Tonight* or *American Idol* for turning us into fame junkies?

Robert Thompson, the director of the Center for the Study of Popular Television at Syracuse University, is one of the nation's foremost experts on celebrity culture. His home office is crammed full of several hundred videotapes, a nineteen-inch Trinitron television set, and five VCRs interconnected by a tangle of cables and splitters. The VCRs all operate on timers, and every evening around eight o'clock—when prime-time television begins—the wilderness of electronics in Thompson's office springs to life. His prime-time recording schedule is never exactly the same. Each week he consults *TV Guide* and sets his VCRs to record the twenty-five hours of television that interest him most. Then, usually once a day, he tears open a bag of Cheetos, hits the PLAY button, and assesses the state of American pop culture.

Thompson is a tall man in his midforties with a florid complexion and a head of wispy brown hair. He dresses casual—jeans and running shoes—and when he talks, he does so with an endearing and sometimes surprising informality, leaning back in his chair with one hand clamped around the back of his head, chatting about the latest episode of *Survivor* or the importance of Super Bowl commercials in pop culture. Thompson lives, breathes, and studies what's on TV, with a commanding sense of purpose. "I watch TV during the day as part of my job, the way my father fixed faucets and water heaters as a plumber," he told me at our first meeting, in his spacious office on campus. "I watched every single episode of *Survivor,* every *Big Brother,* every *Bachelor,* and every *Bachelorettes in Alaska.* A lot of what's on television in America isn't stuff that I would actually choose to watch. But some of it, like *Temptation Island,* I loved."

As it turns out, Thompson was also a fan of my favorite

TV show from childhood. "*Lifestyles of the Rich and Famous* marked the beginning of the television obsession with celebrity lifestyle," he said almost nostalgically. "The show simply gushed. It was all *Isn't this just so wonderful, and wouldn't you love to eat off these gold plates, and drink from these diamond-studded goblets, and go to these parties, and live in these houses?* And the formula worked, because it allowed us to imagine ourselves in their shoes."

During the 1920s and 1930s dozens of "fanzines" fawned over movie stars in a similar manner, but Thompson maintains that these publications and their readers never amounted to much more than a vibrant yet isolated pocket of Americana. In 1923, for example, the best-known magazine about Hollywood celebrities was *Photoplay*. The cover of the October issue that year boasted, "Over 500,000 Circulation." By contrast, in 2005 *People* magazine's circulation was more than seven times as large: over 3.7 million. Nowadays such magazines are supplemented by an array of celebrity-focused television shows like *Entertainment Tonight, Access Hollywood, Cribs,* and virtually everything on the E! network. It is quite possible, Thompson argues, that in the era before World War II, a person living in a small town could go several days without seeing the image of a single celebrity, whereas now it's doubtful that a person in that same town could pass one day without catching a glimpse of Paris Hilton. And in Thompson's view, this trend began around 1984, with Robin Leach.

That era also marked the emergence of cable television. In 1983 the number of U.S. households that subscribed to cable TV totaled 31 million; by 2005 they had surpassed 73 million. Cable made it infinitely easier for entrepreneurs to launch television networks, because they could create a whole range of programming and distribute it nationally without having to build any signal towers. Predictably, programming boomed. In the early 1970s most television viewers had only a few channels to choose from, including the three broadcast networks, PBS, and perhaps one or two independent local stations. By 2005 those viewers had hundreds of choices. According to a 2005 report by the U.S. Department of Labor, this "explosion of programming" is fueling a job growth of 31 percent in the television industry.

The upshot of all this is that the networks on cable—and now satellite as well—need a steady supply of telegenic actors, singers, cooks, talk-show hosts, and meteorologists to fill the increasing number of celebrity slots—or "vacancies," as I will call them. All of this creates a perception, and to some extent a reality, that it is now much easier to become famous. This perception is only bolstered by the emergence of reality TV, which ostensibly makes people famous for simply "being themselves." In fact, so many celebrity vacancies are now being filled by reality-TV "stars" that in the fall of 2005 the annual Casting Data Report of the Screen Actors Guild noted a 10.2 percent decrease in the number of episodic television roles available to its members. The culprit, according to the report, was the rampant growth of reality TV. Unfortunately for SAG members, this shift in the marketplace may be permanent. Mark Andrejevic, of the University of Iowa, the author of *Reality TV: The Work of Being Watched,* argues that reality TV is here to stay. "You have to think of reality TV from an economic standpoint," he says. "The casting is cheap, because the participants aren't paid much, and the shows are easy to make, replicate, and export to other countries around the world. Basically, this is very profitable programming." All this suggests that fame will appear to be increasingly accessible to everyday Americans for the immediate future. As Robert Thompson puts it, "Human beings have had delusions of grandeur since the beginning of time, but now these thoughts no longer seem so delusional. You turn on the TV and there seems to be so much fame to go around."

The increase in celebrity vacancies, combined with the abundance of celebrity-centric programming, may be making an especially strong impression on younger viewers, who often have little perspective on what they are watching. TV can affect children powerfully and in unexpected ways. Perhaps the best recent example comes from September 11, 2001. According to Jim

Greenman, the author of *What Happened to the World?*, footage of the planes crashing into the World Trade Center towers was replayed so often that many children came to believe that dozens of buildings had collapsed. This is hardly the only finding of its kind. According to the *Journal of the American Medical Association*, the typical American youth will have witnessed 40,000 murders and 200,000 other violent acts on television by the time he or she turns eighteen. Admittedly, this is a scary thought. But one also has to wonder, How many viewing hours will be devoted to contests like *American Idol*, in which seemingly every single person in the country is lining up to become famous?

"Any kid who is watching TV, or just paying attention to the world around him, has got to come to the conclusion that being famous brings an awful lot of things that can make your life better," Thompson told me. "After all, do you really have to take the garbage out when you are a Hollywood star? That's why all this celebrity stuff is like catnip for kids."

Apparently "this celebrity stuff" is like catnip for professors as well. The rise of the cable news networks has provided a great many vacancies for academics who are willing to be interviewed on a range of subjects. Hardly a week goes by when Thompson is not called upon to appear on a major television news show to talk about any issue that may be only vaguely related to the history or psychology of television. This attention has prompted Syracuse to give him one of the largest offices on campus, with a panoramic view of rolling green lawns. And the university is in the process of building him an even bigger office, complete with a dressing room.

"My main motivation for doing all these interviews is to extend my classroom, reach a wider audience, and create a broader public discourse," Thompson told me. "But to be honest, I was also probably motivated by the much more raw desire to be acknowledged. And there are times when I'm definitely disturbed by this, and by the fact that these interviews are as important to me as they are. There are times when I find myself counting the hatch marks of how many interviews I've done. I am not someone who ever wanted to give out my autograph or be recognized at the shopping mall—but that doesn't mean I'm not susceptible."

Thompson seems most aware of his own craving for attention during those dry periods when no news organizations call him. In fact, during a subsequent phone conversation he admitted that he was in the midst of a drought. "I haven't had a TV interview since the seventeenth of March, when I was on *Good Morning America* for a taped interview," he told me. "And since then there have been moments when I've gotten worried that my career is over. Of course I'm being a bit hyperbolic—but this stuff is a little like heroin. I guess once you get used to a certain degree of attention, you need more, so you build up a tolerance, and I think there is no end to where this spiral could go . . ."

"But the seventeenth of March was just two weeks ago," I interjected.

"No," Thompson replied gravely. "If it was just two weeks ago, I wouldn't be worried. It was three weeks ago."

Anyone who has ever been in the limelight, even for participating in a high school musical or telling a good story at a cocktail party, can attest to the fact that there is a rush that comes with commanding everyone's attention. Isn't it possible that many behaviors related to fame—including becoming famous, being near the famous, and even reading about the famous—trigger a rush that is potentially addictive?

I eventually paid a visit to Hans Breiter at the Massachusetts General Hospital, in Boston. Breiter is a large teddy bear of a man, well over six feet tall, but with soft facial features and a neatly trimmed red beard. He is one of the nation's top experts on the neurological underpinnings of addiction, and he spends most of his days working in a laboratory equipped with several giant MRI machines. Typically the magnetic fields generated by MRI machines vary in strength by a measure known as a tesla, and you can actually *feel* the difference among the various machines. When you approach the lab's most powerful, seven-tesla machine, for example, you'll sense a slight pull on your feet. This is because the innumerable microscopic pieces of metal embedded in your shoes are gravitating toward the machine's magnet. When I visited the lab, Breiter was guiding a subject into a three-tesla machine. Once the subject slid into this device, he was asked to play a "game of chance" using a small computer screen that showed a spinning roulette wheel. Every time the wheel stopped spinning, the monitor reported how much money the subject had just won or lost. This was "real money," Breiter explained, because after the experiment subjects were allowed to keep their winnings. As this experiment continued, Breiter and his colleagues huddled around another computer screen to see how the subject's brain was reacting to his wins and losses.

Within the past several years Breiter has received a great deal of attention for his research on how our brains react both to "games of chance" and to cocaine use. (He has done another experiment similar to the one I witnessed, in which he gives subjects intravenous infusions of cocaine while they are inside an MRI machine.) He has demonstrated that both activities affect an area of the brain known as the "reward-aversion system." Whenever you feel a rush of either pleasure or pain, that feeling originated in this system. Since the dawn of man the reward-aversion system has played a key role in human evolution. It punishes us with pain when we harm ourselves, and it rewards us with pleasure when we do things that help us survive and reproduce—such as eating and having sex. In addicts this delicate system starts to malfunction. Cocaine users tamper with it by artificially inducing feelings of euphoria; ultimately they succeed in changing the chemistry of their brains, so they need more and more of the drug in order to feel good. Breiter speculated that something similar might occur with gambling. He tested this idea in a relatively simple fashion: when his subjects were in an MRI machine, either gambling or high on cocaine, he asked them to rate how they were feeling. He found that identical parts of the brain "lit up" when gamblers and cocaine users indicated that they were feeling very good. In fact, at such times the MRI scans were so much alike that he could not tell them apart. His studies don't prove that gambling is as addictive as cocaine, but they do suggest that the two affect the brain's circuitry in a remarkably similar fashion.

Although this field of research is still in its infancy, Breiter and others have found the same results when people eat chocolate, view arousing nude pictures, or even play video games. All these activities prompt the brain to release a variety of chemicals or neurotransmitters, including dopamine and endogenous opiates, which ultimately make us feel good. This has led some scientists to observe that the brain is essentially a "giant pharmaceutical factory that manufactures powerful, mind-altering chemicals." Many of us find ourselves craving the activities that trigger these chemical releases. In order to get a fix, we feel driven to eat chocolate constantly, or to bet $1,000 on a Yankees game again and again and again. Indeed, scientists now suspect that a whole range of activities can change the chemistry of some people's brains over time, creating dependencies. One addict's craving for gambling or chocolate may be physiologically as real as another's craving for heroin or nicotine.

Of course, from time to time most of us gamble, or get drunk, or eat too much chocolate. What scientists still don't know is *why* certain people become addicted to these behaviors. According to Alan Marlatt, who runs the Addictive Behaviors Research Center, at the University of Washington, most addicts are looking for a way to "self-medicate." "It is rare to find an addict who is feeling good and just wants to feel a bit better or more euphoric," he told me. "Far more often addicts are trying to escape a low of depression or anxiety." Many clinicians also believe that addicts are looking to exert control over their lives. Craig Nakken, an addiction specialist, argues in his book *Addictive Personality* that when happiness eludes us, and we fall into despair, some of us resort to addictive behaviors that temporarily get us high, change our moods, and offer us relief. The food addict might have a fight with his spouse and then consume several cartons of ice cream. For a moment, instead of feeling depressed and empty, he feels both emotionally and physically full. Again, we all engage in such escapism from time to time, but with addicts these behaviors spiral out of control. True addicts get locked into a destructive cycle in which they come to depend on an activity or a substance for pleasure and comfort. Gradually addicts' priorities—or "value hierarchy"—begin to change, as the addiction becomes more important than work, friends, or family. Eventually, even if addicts desperately want to quit, they find it very difficult to do so.

Nora Volkow, the director of the National Institute for Drug Abuse, says that two things define addiction: whether or not a person can quit, and how well he or she functions in society. For example, we wouldn't say that Bill Gates is "addicted" to making money or being famous, because his desire for these things doesn't appear to debilitate him as a CEO or as a family man. "But if Bill Gates was compulsive about making money or getting fame, at the cost of his integrity, his family, or his health—and he couldn't quit despite wanting to do so—that could be described as an addiction," Volkow told me.

The notion that people can become addicted to a range of substances and activities is gaining credibility not just among clinicians and scientists but with the public as well. Over the past several decades numerous twelve-step recovery groups have emerged, including Alcoholics Anonymous (founded in 1935), Narcotics Anonymous (circa 1950), Gamblers Anonymous (1957), Overeaters Anonymous (1960), Debtors Anonymous (1968), Sex Addicts Anonymous (1977), Clutterers Anonymous (1989), Shoplifters Anonymous (1992), and On-Line Gamers Anonymous (2002).

As far as I know, there are no support groups catering to the celebrity-obsessed niches I explored—no Attention Seekers Anonymous, Celebrity Sidekicks Anonymous, or Die-hard Fans Anonymous. This may seem like a silly notion, but if some people are getting hooked on the rush of shoplifting or playing video games, isn't it possible that others are getting high by fawning over celebrities or, better yet, by joining their entourages and riding with them in their limos? Isn't it even more likely that a select few are getting high by receiving enormous amounts of attention from hordes of cheering fans? Don't all these activities offer at least a bit of euphoria and a certain degree of transcendence or escapism? So why couldn't they be addictive?

The final and perhaps most important issue to consider is availability. Many health care experts, including those at the National Institutes of Health, believe that one of the leading causes of alcoholism may be how readily available alcohol is. Similarly, there is a growing belief that gambling addictions are on the rise, in large part, because of the spread of casinos. Craig Nakken writes, "The more available addictive objects and events are, the greater the number of people who form addictive relationships with them." Wouldn't this apply to fame? If cable television and reality TV have helped increase the availability of fame, and if fame itself is addictive, might this explain why so many people are pining for it? And couldn't the same logic apply to celebrity watching? If celebrity tabloids and TV shows are so readily available, and perhaps even mildly addictive, might this not explain why we can never get enough of them? In the final analysis, could many of us be suffering from a widespread and insidious addiction that no one has ever bothered to diagnose?

Of course, one has to wonder whether other factors, too—including parenting, neurobiology, education, technology, and even evolution—are shaping the way we think about fame and famous people. Perhaps the juggernaut of celebrity is really a combination of many forces, converging like disparate weather systems to form a single, massive storm. This book is a study of that storm—both in terms of how it comes together and how it plays out within the three niches I've identified.

As I set out to write this book, my most immediate concern was my own objectivity. I quickly realized that writing about fame makes it nearly impossible to remain clear-eyed and grounded.

To begin with, whatever you say is bound to rev up the very machine you are "objectively" trying to investigate. You can critique or observe celebrity all you want, but in the end you are just adding to the frenzy. And you have to question your own motives every step of the way, because the mere act of observing and commenting on fame can turn into a vehicle for making yourself famous. While I was writing my first book, much of which focused on poor and middle-class people living in such dangerous places as flood plains and fire corridors, my phone never rang. But in the early stages of this book I did a very brief commentary for National Public Radio in which I talked about Michael Jackson. The next day my phone was ringing off the hook. I'd be lying if I said I didn't enjoy this on some level. In fact, I'd be lying if I told you that I didn't consider doing another commentary on Michael Jackson. Robert Thompson was right: there *is* something addictive about this stuff. The poet Rainer Rilke was quite prescient when he observed that anyone who investigates the "thousands of fame-wheels and fame-belts" of the fame industry is "ultimately also pressed into service and soon contributes to the machine's monstrous actions and berserk roaring." I tried to acknowledge these two things and bear them in mind throughout the writing of this book.

Another pitfall for me was my background. I quickly realized that who I was—namely, a non-television-watching, parka-wearing, nonfiction-writing, generally unslick guy from Buffalo, New York—was a bit of a disadvantage. That said, I also think my role as an outsider helped me. The fact that I wrote books—rather than screenplays or television shows or snippets for *TV Guide*—often put people at ease. "I usually don't do interviews," one high-powered Hollywood manager told me. "But no one reads books anymore, so I suppose it can't hurt talking to you."

Finally, it's worth noting that it was my status as Buffalonian, oddly enough, that opened the door to my first niche, the world of aspiring celebrities. One day, while I was leafing through the *Sports Illustrated* swimsuit issue, something other than the scantily clad beauties caught my eye. It was a single word: the name of my beloved hometown, to be precise. Alongside models hailing from Brazil, Argentina, and Nigeria was a Buffalo girl named Jessica White. I was surprised for several reasons, starting with the fact that I couldn't recall a single memory of a woman in a string bikini during my eighteen years of growing up in Buffalo. But seeing Jessica White in these pages was no fluke. This was her third year posing for *Sports Illustrated,* and she was, by all accounts, well on her way to becoming a supermodel.

Curious to learn more about her, I visited the *Sports Illustrated* Web site, which said, "At fourteen Jessica thumbed through Buffalo's Yellow Pages looking for modeling schools. Less than twelve months later she signed with the prestigious IMG Models of New York City." I was intrigued. How exactly did one go from the Buffalo Yellow Pages to stardom in less than a year? Such a path seemed both improbable and random. But as I soon discovered, it was neither.

PART I

THE WORLD OF ASPIRING

CHILD CELEBRITIES

Going to Fame School

LOOKING FOR aspiring celebrities in America is a little like looking for dehydrated nomads at a desert encampment— they are everywhere, and their thirst is so intense it's almost palpable. So when it came to finding places inhabited by fame seekers, I had plenty of options. I eventually decided to focus on young people—the kids and early teens of the "reality-TV generation," who grew up in the 1990s watching *The Real World* and other shows that seem to offer everyone at least fifteen minutes of fame. I believed, rightly or wrongly, that kids were more likely to give me emotionally honest answers about why they wanted to become famous. And for some reason I felt a lot of sympathy for kids who yearned to become famous that frankly, hard as I tried, I simply couldn't muster for adults who wanted the same thing. All this persuaded me that what I really needed was a school of sorts—an academy for aspiring celebrities—and as it so happens I found just such a place right in my own hometown.

I didn't realize it at the time, but when I was growing up, Buffalo's doorway into the world of fame and glamour was on the same street as my elementary school. If I had only traveled a bit farther down Harlem Road, heading south toward the Mount Calvary Cemetery and a bleak stretch of strip malls that housed (and still house) an odd smattering of such businesses as the Buffalo Gun Center, Tony's Pizza, and Stylin' Tat-2, Tattoo & Body Piercing. In the midst of this drab suburban sprawl, I might have noticed a white house with conspicuous, bright-purple trim and a sign reading Personal Best.

This hub for would-be stars is run by Susan Makai, who in her heyday, in the mid-1970s, was the closest thing Buffalo had to an A-list celebrity. After winning the title of Miss Buffalo in the early stages of the 1974 Miss America Pageant, she became the region's first female TV meteorologist and one of the first unmarried cheerleaders to join the ranks of the Buffalo Jills. In the twilight of her stardom Makai was known informally as the "Movie Lady," because she introduced a new movie each night at eight o'clock on Channel 29. Makai took her job seriously and she spoke at length about how each film was conceived, cast, and shot—and she did so in an accessible, upbeat way, almost like a well-spoken neighbor who happens to be a film buff.

During her tenure as the Movie Lady, Makai began working for the local branch of John Robert Powers, or JRP. At its core, JRP is a cross between an acting school and a talent agency. It is a place where children and teenagers can learn to walk like fashion models, practice reading scripts, and perhaps meet a bona fide Hollywood or New York agent. From a strictly business perspective, JRP functions like McDonald's: owners of a franchise use the company's name and patented formula to open new branches and make money. The company has grown steadily over the past half century, and JRP now operates in at least thirty states and a number of countries around the globe, from England to Indonesia and Vietnam.

JRP is hardly the only business of its kind. Dozens of other modeling and acting schools across the country, including Barbizon and John Casablanca, have created a fast-growing and lucrative industry. Many of these schools have proved quite resourceful at recruitment. Representatives from Barbizon persuaded several public schools in Montgomery County, Maryland, to let them give talks during class time about the ins and outs of the modeling industry. Students were asked to submit their contact information if they wanted to learn more about modeling or become eligible to win a college scholarship. Several days later parents around the county received telephone calls from Barbizon salespeople who explained that their children had expressed an interest in modeling and that they could purchase six weeks' worth of lessons for just $1,800. Soon afterward Montgomery County banned Barbizon from its schools. Apparently, however, this hasn't set much of a precedent elsewhere. According to Ed Beaky, who has owned and run the Barbizon school in Dallas, Texas, for decades, it is standard practice for his employees to visit public schools and recruit students during the school day.

Of all the modeling schools now in operation, JRP is certainly among the oldest and most reputable. It was conceived in 1923 by John Robert Powers, a failed actor turned businessman. He designed a curriculum and wrote several books that offered a comprehensive strategy on how to become a successful model. In his 1960 classic, *How to Have Model Beauty, Poise, & Personality,* the author's biographical note reads, "John Robert Powers has advised, met, admired and observed more women than any other man in history. His practiced eye perceives the women who come to the John Robert Powers Modeling Agency not as they are, but as the beautiful, charming creatures they could—and should—be."

Powers's book is full of brief chapters with titles like "Tips on Training Your Eyes to Sparkle," "9 Ways to Put Charm in Your Voice," "How to Buy a Hat," and "Teenage Skin Problems." At its best, the advice Powers offers is commonsensical; at its worst, it's asinine. In his section on "Teenage Skin Problems," for example, he has this to say: "Protruding nose hair can be clipped occasionally with a scissors but must never be pulled. Death has actually resulted from tweezing this area." The book's overall theme is that women must always strive for beauty and glamour. "It is a woman's birthright to be attractive and charming," Powers writes. "In a sense, it is her duty as well . . . She is the bowl of flowers on the table of life." The path to glamour, he asserts, is open to everyone—no matter who she is or what she looks like: "There are no problems which cannot be solved if they are simply treated as problems instead of unchangeable drawbacks.

Some flaws can be corrected—others can be made to fade away in the light of other perfected charms. Girls with buck teeth have become movie stars. Grandmothers have become glamour girls. The least pretty girls have become the most popular." As proof of how easily attainable beauty and charm can be, Powers offers the example of a girl he once met who had a debilitating stutter. He quickly diagnosed the root of the problem and offered a solution: "One day I casually suggested a change in her hair style and gave her lipstick to experiment with. . . . Gradually as the days went along, I saw the metamorphis [sic] of this shy sensitive girl into a beautiful young lady. She saw the changes, too— and at the end of a few weeks she no longer stuttered!"

Powers took the concept of the traditional finishing school, added a healthy dollop of Dale Carnegie–style self-empowerment, and threw in some quick training on how to act and pose for the camera. After just a few classes his students could acquire manners, heightened confidence, and the know-how to become budding stars. In theory, a successful JRP student could—if she followed each prescribed step—completely reinvent herself, à la Jay Gatsby. "Modeling has changed the lives of thousands of Powers Girls," wrote Powers. "Small town girls have become leaders of New York society. A cantor's daughter from the lower East Side became the editor of a top fashion magazine. A barge captain's daughter married into royalty. One girl married an ambassador. Another married the head of one of our largest corporations. Others have married Hollywood producers, Broadway directors, famous actors."

His approach rapidly proved a success. According to the JRP Web site, Powers's original school, in New York City, attracted droves of students, and the agency it spawned went on to represent such stars as Ava Gardner, Barbara Stanwyck, Lucille Ball, and Henry Fonda in their early modeling careers. In subsequent years the JRP schools trained thousands of students around the country—Diana Ross, Raquel Welch, and Jacqueline Kennedy among them—and cemented a reputation as the definitive conduit for aspiring stars of all varieties.

The common denominator at the heart of JRP's success, the golden carrot that keeps students coming, seems to be the promise of fame. Time and again during my research I met kids from all over the country who told me some version of the same story. They were driving with their parents, or sitting in their bedrooms, when they heard an ad on the radio asking if they wanted to be famous. The ads varied from state to state, but the basic pitch was always the same: "You could be the next big star!"

In fairness to these fame schools, their sales pitches are not outright scams. At some point JRP students generally do get a chance to meet talent agents from New York and Hollywood. But here's the rub: this usually happens only when the students pay an additional fee of several thousand dollars to attend an independently operated pageant or "talent convention," where thousands of participants compete against one another for the attention of several dozen agents and managers from New York and L.A. And technically, the only way to get invited to a talent convention like this is to attend a registered acting or modeling school like the ones operated by John Robert Powers.

Susan Makai started working for the JRP School in Buffalo in 1983. At the time, the school's owner, a local businessman named Jim Satterfield, needed someone to run it, and Makai seemed the perfect candidate for the job. Her various stints as Miss Buffalo, the TV meteorologist, and Channel 29's Movie Lady had given her the visibility and the experience to speak with authority about celebrityhood—albeit within the somewhat limited setting of the Rust Belt. Makai also had a master's degree in education, which qualified her as a teacher. The only problem was the cost of tuition. A typical course at JRP has never been cheap. "Even back in the early 1980s they were charging twelve hundred dollars for a course that was just a few months long," Makai told me. "And that's a lot of money to ask from people in a market like Buffalo." This was especially true in the early eighties, when the region was rapidly slipping into economic depression. Not surprisingly, within a few years the Buffalo branch of JRP closed its doors for good.

After the school closed, Makai immediately began receiving calls from former students who were still interested in taking classes. Several of them even volunteered to work for her for free in exchange for classes. Eventually Makai became convinced that she could open up her own low-budget, mom-and-pop version of the JRP School. She would offer similar training in fine manners and the basics of acting—and her students would still ultimately have a chance to attend a talent convention—but Makai would charge markedly less for her classes. One of the areas in which Makai cut costs was advertising. There would be no elaborate radio campaigns selling the dream of fame, which Makai had never felt comfortable with anyway. Instead she would do things the Buffalo way, which meant taking out a small ad in the phone book and then relying on word of mouth.

During the 1990s Makai slowly built a reputation in Buffalo as a fair businesswoman who genuinely cared about her students. But things didn't really take off for her until 1998, when a fourteen-year-old African American girl named Jessica White walked through the door. White attended several classes at Personal Best and then traveled with Makai and a handful of other students to a talent convention in New York run by the International Modeling and Talent Association (IMTA). There, in mid-July of 1999, as White mingled with hundreds of other children and teenagers from all over the country, the improbable happened: she landed a contract with IMG Models.

From that moment on Jessica White's rise was meteoric. She traveled to Milan, Paris, and back to New York, walking the runway for DKNY, Kenneth Cole, Chloe, and Sonia Rykiel. Jessica's mother, Fanny White, could not get time off from work to go on many of these trips, so Susan Makai often served as her "mother agent"—a long-standing position in the industry to help models too young to travel and negotiate on their own. Typically, a big agency like IMG will take 20 percent of a model's income in return for finding her work; then, a mother agent will collect an additional 5 to 10 percent. The experience was eye-opening for Makai. "I didn't know what the world was like on that level," she told me. "I'd never even heard of Jean Paul Gaultier."

White soon began appearing in countless magazines, including *Vogue, Harper's Bazaar, Seventeen, Teen, Jane, Teen Vogue, Elle,* and, perhaps most noticeably, the *Sports Illustrated* swimsuit issues of 2003, 2004, and 2005. Needless to say, this kind of press was far more valuable to Personal Best than any amount of advertising on a local radio station. Back in Buffalo word quickly spread through an informal yet vast network of hairdressers, church groups, and portrait photographers that the best path to stardom was not a reality-TV show but a local thoroughfare called Harlem Road, on which sat a small white two-story house with bright-purple trim.

I paid my first visit to Personal Best on a cold Thursday evening, as a light waft of lake-effect snow shot skyward in spiraling eddies. The sides of Harlem Road were fortified with embankments of snow and ice as high as five feet in some places, the color of which had long since been blackened with the grime of the mud-splattered pavement. I parked my car on a lonely side street, where a long row of identical tan-brick ranch houses and skeletal trees stretched toward the horizon. In the distance dogs were barking as if to ward off the cold.

As I stepped through the front door of Personal Best, I came into a bright waiting room painted in flamboyant shades of pink and purple and furnished with a few chairs and three metal magazine racks: one for *People* magazine, one for *Us Weekly,* and one for *Elle.* No one was in sight, so I cleared my throat to announce myself, and suddenly Susan Makai popped her head through a doorway. She was older, and a little blonder than I remembered from her Movie Lady days, but the contours of her face and the bubbly energy of her voice were familiar.

Makai greeted me, tossed me a copy of the most recent *Sports Illustrated* swimsuit issue, and then excused herself to do some last-minute preparations for an upcoming meeting. This meeting, she told me, was intended for her more advanced students—those who had already completed an eight-week "personal development course" in which they learned how to look, talk, and carry themselves in public. The first class, for example, taught the basics of posture and poise. The second covered how to walk properly and project a positive attitude. The third focused on nail care, skin care, general health, and the use of makeup. The fourth offered tips on choosing a wardrobe, wearing the right colors, and how best to shop. Many of Makai's advanced students had also taken Personal Best courses in the fundamentals of acting and public speaking.

Tonight Makai was offering an information session for those students interested in joining the school's annual trip to the IMTA convention in New York City—the same convention where Jessica White had been discovered. Students who wanted to make the trip would have to devote the next six months to learning monologues, fine-tuning their posture, buying the right clothing, and raising an average of $3,000 for the cost of attending.

At around six o'clock thirteen of Makai's students began arriving and heading to the back of the house, where a former living room had been converted into a performance space with two dozen or so folding chairs and a number of glaring overhead lights. The students were all female, ranging in age from eight to twenty, and without exception they wore chic outfits that included pearls, Guess scarves, and Ugg sheepskin boots. The parents who accompanied them were strikingly unhip by comparison, and rather unapologetic about it. Clearly hard-working, solidly middle-class Buffalonians, they included a retired police officer, a town clerk, an elementary school secretary, a toolmaker, a bus-parts salesman, a worker at a turbo-compressor plant, and the proprietor of a golf driving range and hot dog stand. None of them struck me as the sort of people who would lightly toss away $3,000.

Eventually Makai emerged from her office, called the meeting to order, and asked the students to introduce themselves. The first to do so was the oldest, Sarah Hornbrick, who said matter-of-factly, "My name is Sarah. I am twenty years old, I recently graduated from Buffalo State College, I now manage an apartment complex, and I want to be famous." The other girls nodded politely, and Sarah sat down. Moments later a four-teen-year-old girl named Lucinda Wells rose to her feet and explained that she hoped to become a movie star. In her hands she was clutching a large three-ring binder emblazoned with the words I WANT TO BE FAMOUS.

Over the following days I interviewed Lucinda Wells and virtually every other girl in attendance that night, and our chats were generally dominated by talk of fame. Many of the girls plainly wanted celebrityhood, but when I asked *why*, they were often at a loss. "You can ask anyone in my family or any of my friends, and they will tell you that what I want more than anything is to become famous," Lucinda told me. When I pressed her on the matter, she added emphatically, "It's just what I want to do. It's the one thing that makes me feel good about myself."

The most obvious draw for many of the girls was the glamour that comes with fame—a point that one mother made quite vociferously. Her daughter had said, "For me, it is not even about the glitz and glamour. . . ." when her mother quickly interjected, "Yes, it is! She loves being pampered. She loves someone doing her nails. She loves someone rubbing lotion on her face and feet. And she likes the attention. She's a brat!" The girl, who seemed somewhat shocked, confessed to me rather sheepishly, "I'm a princess. It's not my fault. My mom always told me, 'Always shine, never blend.'"

For a number of girls fame also meant a one-way ticket out of Buffalo. Sixteen-year-old Amy Lumber, an aspiring actress, told me that Personal Best—like a number of out-of-town colleges she was investigating—offered her an escape from her father, who could be verbally abusive. She didn't need to be a movie star, she told me. "I could do commercials. Like this one for Listerine." She then recited an entire Listerine commercial and shot me a hopeful glance.

Most of the girls at Personal Best appeared to be quite excited about the possibility of leaving Buffalo and moving out to Hollywood. For the most part, they seemed to have formed their impressions of Hollywood and the "realities" of being a celebrity by watching *Entertainment Tonight* and *Access Hollywood.* Sarah Hornbrick and a few others acknowledged that these shows were probably not entirely accurate—but this made little difference to Sarah. "I realize that they cut out all the dry parts," she told me. "But it still seems like a pretty good life." Other girls had come to this conclusion simply by watching TV shows that were set in Los Angeles. "I hate Buffalo—it's so cold," Lucinda Wells told me. "I want to live in L.A. From what I've seen on *MTV News,* it just looks so exciting."

It is worth noting that, according to our survey of middle school students in Rochester, teenagers who regularly watch certain celebrity-focused TV shows—*Entertainment Tonight, Access Hollywood,* and *The Insider*—are more likely than others to believe that they themselves will be famous someday. The same appears to be true for teenagers who read magazines like *Us Weekly, Star, People, Teen People, YM,* and *J-14.* There is also a strong correlation between how many hours of television teenagers watch and how badly they want to become famous. One of the survey questions was "If you could push a magic button that would change your life in one way, which of the following would you pick?" The options were "(a) Becoming smarter"; "(b) Becoming much bigger or stronger"; "(c) Becoming famous"; "(d) Becoming beautiful or more beautiful"; and "(e) My life doesn't need any improving." Among those teens who watched one hour or less of TV a day, only 15 percent of the boys and 17 percent of the girls chose fame. But among those who watched five hours or more a day—and many did—29 percent of the boys and 37 percent of the girls chose fame.

Admittedly, it's unclear whether TV is to blame or whether the kids are watching these shows because they already believe they're destined for fame. There is evidence, however, that some TV shows are to blame. Another survey question was "When you watch TV shows or read magazine articles about the lives of celebrities, how do they make you feel?" A number of teens commented that such stories made them feel they could and would become famous. One wrote, "They make me feel like one day I will probably be in their shoes." Another wrote: "They make me feel like one day I'll be there on the magazine, talking or telling people about my life."

The girls at Personal Best said that their single most important motivator was not TV but the indisputable fact that Jessica White—a regular girl from Buffalo—had once sat in this same schoolroom, gone off to this same talent convention, and ultimately become famous. Perhaps no one was more acutely aware of this than Susan Makai, who found herself in the difficult position of touting White's success—something she had to do in order to keep students coming to her school—while trying to temper her students' expectations. "I have to walk a very fine line," Makai later told me. And this is precisely what she tried to do at the meeting that Thursday evening.

"Jessica White is the most successful model to ever come out of Personal Best," Makai told her students. "But her situation is rare. So just remember, you are taking a chance. You are rolling the dice." Despite this admonition and all the seemingly obvious logic behind it, almost every one of the girls later told me she believed that she had at least a 50 percent chance of being discovered and becoming a star. Many of them had already begun to plan a move to Los Angeles, and some were being pressured for gifts from the money they would supposedly earn in the future. Fifteen-year-old Kim Palazzo told me with a shy smile, "My dad wants a Corvette, my neighbor wants a Harley, my brother wants a helicopter, my mom wants a '68 Camaro, and my track coach wants me to build the school an indoor track."

Toward the end of the evening Makai broached the subject of money. The attendance fee for the New York convention is set by the IMTA, which refuses to disclose the amount. Above and beyond this, Personal Best and other schools are free to add their own fees in order to make a profit. Makai charges a minimum of $2,850, which covers the attendance fee, airfare, lodging, and a dozen or so classes at Personal Best to prepare for the convention. (As I would later learn, Makai's prices are positively cheap compared with those of other talent schools, some of which charge almost twice as much.) The IMTA also imposes a number of other fees. Parents who want to watch their kids perform must pay $395 apiece to enter the premises. (And of course they must pay for their own hotel and airfare.) The IMTA also hosts an official luncheon and an official dinner, each of which costs roughly $100 per person. Finally, headshots, makeup, clothing, and all meals must be paid for out of pocket. All told, many of the Personal Best parents would be spending $5,000—an awful lot of money for a middle-class family in Buffalo. I assumed that many of the parents would have serious reservations. To my surprise, however, not a single parent raised any concerns or objections. The same was true later on, when I spoke with parents privately. They simply assumed that a shot at fame, like a college education, came at a high price. At times I had to bite my tongue. One girl asked during our interview if I could recommend a good SAT preparation class. I recommended the Princeton Review, which costs about $900. Days later I learned that the girl's parents—who had already promised to set aside roughly $7,000 for her to attend the IMTA convention in 2005 and again in 2006—rejected the Princeton Review as too costly.

My initial reaction to all this was some combination of shock and puzzlement. One of the things I had always valued about Buffalo was that it was inhabited by down-to-earth people. As my father loved to point out with pride, this was the self-proclaimed "City of No Illusions." So what was going on?

For one thing, the IMTA offered a prize that was unavailable anywhere in or near Buffalo: a chance at becoming a celebrity. Maybe if Buffalo were situated on the outskirts of Los Angeles, where agents and managers are ubiquitous, the city's residents wouldn't be so eager to shell out this kind of money. But in the heart of the Rust Belt fame was a rare commodity. And the IMTA convention would provide more than just a shot at becoming rich and famous: it offered a bite-size taste of the glamour that New York City had to offer. After all, this convention wasn't being held at the Holiday Inn in Newark, where it would have cost far less. It was being held at the Hilton Hotel on Sixth Avenue in midtown Manhattan, just a stone's throw from Carnegie Hall and Radio City Music Hall. IMTA organizers readily admitted that this was deliberate. "Families turn this into a vacation for themselves," the association's chief operating officer, Nancy Mancuso, explained to me. "These families come with their kids, parents, grandparents, and guests so they can experience it as well." Even by modest estimates, a family of four attending an IMTA convention in New York or Los Angeles could easily spend $10,000 when the costs of airfare, hotel, wardrobe, headshots, entrance fees, dinners, luncheons, and prior acting classes were tallied. "I don't know how these families do it," Mancuso said.

"I have never been to New York City before," a mother named Rosa Polowska told me after the Thursday-evening meeting. "We're from the little town of East Aurora, and for us even going into downtown Buffalo is a big deal. So this is a big trip—it's scary—but we'll be with Susan, so she'll know what to do."

"I think it's going to be a great experience!" added the woman's eight-year-old daughter, Jodi, the youngest of the thirteen girls going on the trip.

"What if someone notices you and you get to be on TV?" her mother asked.

"You just gave me the chills," Jodi replied. Then she smiled, shrugged, and added, "I am just looking forward to seeing a real Broadway musical and going up in an airplane for the first time. I want to get a window seat, because you are so high up, and I want to be able to look down and see things, even if we are just going through clouds."

In the world of adolescent psychology at least two theories shed light on why so many teenagers are prone to believe they are destined to live exceptional, celebrity-like lives. Both theories first appeared in 1967, in a groundbreaking paper by a psychologist named David Elkind. Elkind maintains that by their very nature, adolescents are unable to grasp what other people are thinking or feeling, so they exist in a sort of egocentric daze, assuming that everyone else is as obsessed with their lives as they are. He articulates this notion in his Imaginary Audience theory, which posits that teens often feel as if they were on a grand stage in front of a watchful audience that noticed every facet of their appearance and behavior. Hence the teenage drama queen. Her bad hair day is a catastrophe because she believes that everyone she encounters is watching only her. And because this teenager feels that she is of such importance to so many people, she comes to believe that her feelings and her life must be utterly unique. This leads to Elkind's second theory, known simply as the Personal Fable, in which an adolescent believes that his or her destiny is special and that conventional rules or odds don't apply. Hence the teen daredevil who shrugs off the dangers of drag racing, or the aspiring starlet who goes to an IMTA convention utterly convinced that she has at least a 50 percent chance of being discovered. The belief underlying both these theories is that teenagers—for both social and biological reasons—are predisposed to having daily delusions of grandeur in which they feel as if they are playing the lead in epic movies about themselves.

To test these theories psychologists have devised the Imaginary Audience Scale, which involves a written test with twelve different scenarios. One scenario asks the subject to imagine that he or she just got a bad haircut and then offers three options for coping with it: "going out and not worrying about my hair"; "sitting where people won't notice me much"; or simply "staying home." Results from this and similar tests indicate that young adolescents are far more self-conscious than older adolescents or adults. Admittedly, one problem with these findings is that the older subjects may be lying, or at least moderating their responses, in order to give more mature-sounding or socially desirable answers. After all, how many forty-year-old men would readily admit to wanting to hide after an especially bad haircut? But in general the results do seem to reinforce the notion that most young teens are emotionally charged, insecure, and extremely self-centered.

Some psychologists, including Daniel Lapsley, of Ball State University, believe that this isn't really such a bad thing. According to Lapsley, both the imaginary audience and the personal fable are natural parts of the daydreaming that goes on during the so-called "separation-individuation" process. This process generally occurs as adolescents start to form relationships and define themselves outside the family unit. Daydreaming can be an important coping mechanism during this period, Lapsley says, because it allows adolescents to conjure fantasies in which they assert themselves as individuals. These are painless trial runs in which they can visualize doing bold things within the safe confines of their imaginations. A girl like Lucinda Wells may never become the starlet she yearns to be—in reality, she may not even command much of an audience in her high school cafeteria—but by imagining herself as a celebrity within the context of her surroundings, she starts to carve out a unique identity for herself as a mature adult.

One has to wonder, though, whether pop culture is affecting this normal maturation process. For example, what kind of impact is *Teen People* or *Us Weekly* having on Lucinda Wells's daydreaming? For that matter, what kind of impact is reality TV, or all the celebrity vacancies on cable television, having on teens? And what about businesses like the John Robert Powers schools and the IMTA conventions, which promise to turn these distant fantasies into reality? It seems reasonable to assume that all these factors that make fame seem so accessible actually reinforce or even prolong a teen's use of the imaginary audience and the personal fable. According to Lapsley, "The danger is that if these adolescents don't curb all this daydreaming with a healthy dose of reality, they could end up in relationships that are manipulative or exploitive. Basically, after spending so much time in front of an imaginary audience, they might ultimately only be interested in forming relationships that serve their need to be admired, instead of forming ones that authentically engage other people."

Sadly, studies show that the imaginary-audience phenomenon increases significantly among adolescents who feel neglected by their parents. One such study, which was conducted among 251 seventh-graders in the Midwest, showed that adolescent girls who felt their parents had rejected them scored significantly higher on the Imaginary Audience Scale than those who didn't. A rather obvious interpretation of these results is that kids who don't get much support or attention at home are likely to fantasize about getting it elsewhere. And why merely fantasize about it when you might actually make it happen at an *American Idol* tryout or an IMTA convention?

Perhaps the most difficult issue to consider is causation: What makes adolescents so vulnerable to lapses in reason and delusions of grandeur? One explanation is that they haven't acquired enough life experience to put everything in its proper perspective. Yet according to many scientists, some compelling biological explanations may also exist. They believe that adolescents' adrenal glands, which secrete hormones, become active almost a decade before their brains are fully capable of exercising mature judgment and rational thought. In fact, one of the last parts of the brain to develop is the prefrontal cortex, which governs logic. According to Laurence Steinberg, of Temple University, one of the nation's preeminent adolescent psychologists, it all comes down to timing. Steinberg describes the part of the brain that controls judgment and rational thought as an "executive suite" that gradually comes "online" over the course of adolescence. He concludes that the gap in time between the onset of puberty and the full activation of the executive suite creates the "special vulnerability and challenge of adolescence."

Steinberg's argument appears to have direct implications for teenagers like Lucinda Wells. If Lucinda was, in fact, more biologically vulnerable to lapses in rational thought and surges of feeling, then was she not also more vulnerable to sales pitches that were thin on logic and heavy on the promise of big emotional payoffs? John Robert Powers proclaimed, "Girls with buck teeth have become movie stars. . . . The least pretty girls have become the most popular." To my adult brain these promises seem pretty suspect. But if I were a teenager, and the logic circuitry in my brain was not fully developed, might I, too, not beg my parents for $3,000? Might I not develop a personal fable, dismiss the long odds, and tell myself that I had a 50 percent chance of making it? Perhaps it isn't that teenagers are addicted to fame as much as that they are biologically predisposed to crave what fame promises: endless amounts of attention.

I made a point of talking to almost every one of the thirteen Personal Best girls who were bound for the IMTA convention in New York. My most telling encounter by far was with Amy Lumber, the aspiring Listerine spokeswoman. I met with Amy several times at a coffee shop near Personal Best, and eventually she invited me to visit her home in the town of Elma, just outside Buffalo. It was late dusk when I neared her house. As I pulled into the driveway, my headlights illuminated a small herd of deer next to the rusted carcass of a 1936 Ford. The deer hesitated for a split second, as if reluctant to leave their find, and then scattered into the night shadows.

The Lumbers' property contained roughly a dozen cars in various conditions, ranging from immobile wrecks like the old Ford on the front lawn to pristine classics that looked as if they'd been preserved in a museum for the past thirty years. Amy's father, Rudolph Lumber, was a retired U.S. Army captain who now devoted much of his time to restoring old cars. Amy had little interest in her father's passion. She had more pressing matters to worry about. In fact, she'd made this point quite clear to me during our chats at the coffee shop.

Amy was a short girl with moss-green eyes and a mane of bright-red hair. She spoke quickly and tended to sigh heavily, as if she was under considerable stress. "I already feel that I am falling behind for my age group," she said. "I feel like the world is advancing rapidly, and there are so many kids who are doing amazing things. Like when you turn on *Oprah,* you see kids who have sold paintings for millions, made scientific discoveries, or recorded songs by age eleven. I even saw a girl who is so good at the stock market that she'll be able to retire by the age of twenty-five."

One of Amy's goals in life was to become famous, though she insisted that she was not interested in a measly fifteen minutes of fame. She wanted the lasting variety—the sort that is inextricably linked with great achievement. Amy's biggest fear, she told me, was that her teenage years would slip away and she would somehow fail to make a name for herself. "I am more afraid of failing than I am of death," she said. When I asked her where this fear came from, her reply came swiftly: "My father— no matter what I am doing, he'll push me to do more. I think the army made him a little crazy."

When I arrived at her house, Amy welcomed me with the impeccable manners of a debutante, taking my coat, pouring me a drink, and offering me a tour of the house. Her red hair swayed from side to side as she chatted pleasantly and escorted me through the living room, the dining room, and the kitchen before asking me if I cared to see the basement. "My father has a lot of World War II memorabilia down there," she explained. "I thought that might interest you."

We descended a narrow staircase and emerged into an enormous, museumlike room, lined with a number of small alcoves and glass display cases. The entire far end of the room was dedicated to Rudolph Lumber's World War II memorabilia—uniforms, medals, photographs. What immediately caught my eye, however, was a large space at the front of the room, which was set up as a shrine to Marilyn Monroe. Along with numerous books, photographs, and figurines were some more unusual items—including a life-size replica of Monroe complete with an attached fan that blew up her skirt, simulating the famous scene from *The Seven Year Itch.* Yet by far the most striking aspect of this display was what Amy referred to as the "off-limits section," where several mannequins were dressed in clothing that Monroe had once actually worn—a strapless evening gown, a terry-cloth bathrobe, a pair of high heels, and a sexy black nightgown.

"Who does all this stuff belong to?" I asked finally.

"My father," Amy replied. "I think it's a little spooky, don't you? We finally got him to put the mannequins in the basement. They used to be up on the first floor, and sometimes you'd bump into them in the middle of the night."

When I asked Amy why her father was so taken with Marilyn Monroe, she shrugged and offered only a blank look. Later, when the subject arose again, Amy's mother said, "I guess he's just infatuated with pretty movie stars." Amy nodded. As Mrs. Lumber straightened up the kitchen, she went on to explain that she herself collected Elvis paraphernalia—albeit not with the same fervor as her husband. Her collection, for example, did not contain anything of value or have an "off-limits section."

Eventually Rudolph Lumber wandered into the kitchen and introduced himself. He was a strapping man, well over six feet tall, with a horseshoe of hair that framed a gleaming bald spot. Both his daughter and his wife visibly stiffened when he entered the room. I made a lame attempt at breaking the ice by expressing interest in his Marilyn Monroe nightgown.

"You're not going to write about the location of this house, are you?" he asked curtly. "Because some of the items in my collection are pretty valuable." I quickly replied that I would say nothing about the exact location of the house, because I didn't want to be responsible for any cat burglars snooping around. "Good," Lumber said gruffly. "Because I don't want to be responsible for shooting them."

Our conversation was mercifully cut short by the arrival of the fourth and final member of the family: Amy's nineteen-year-old sister, Barbara. Barbara was a spark plug of a girl with a brash, raspy voice. A squawking, fuzzy little chick sat on her shoulder. "This is my pet," she explained. "I want to be able to ride around with this little guy on my shoulder as if I were a pirate or something."

"If it starts crowing at dawn, I'm reaching for my gun," Lumber warned.

"Whatever," Barbara said.

When I looked at Lumber to see how he had taken this brush-off, he was smiling. In fact, from the moment Barbara walked in the door, his mood seemed to improve. Before long he was bragging to me about her exploits as one of the area's top drag racers. "She's a chip off the old block," he gushed. "Did I mention that she has broken into the twelves? She did a quarter of a mile from a standing start in the twelve-second range! And she did it in a street car with no modifications."

Lumber rambled on about Barbara's racing exploits, and as he did, a rather obvious conclusion dawned on me: each of his daughters had taken up one of his passions. Barbara was a budding drag racer and car aficionado, while Amy was striving to become a Hollywood starlet. Later on, when we had a moment alone, I asked Amy if she thought her father's interest in Marilyn Monroe had any bearing on her desire to become famous. "Maybe," she replied tentatively. "When something sticks with you through your whole life, it tends to have an effect on you—no matter what way you look at it."

Perhaps what impressed me most about Amy Lumber was her seriousness of purpose. "In order to be remembered or to achieve something—that doesn't start when you're adult, it starts now," she told me. "It's just like Benjamin Franklin. He was a millionaire by the time he was a teenager." Amy seemed to believe that her dream of becoming famous would depend almost entirely on how hard she worked. In this regard she is actually quite typical of American kids. Teenagers in the Rochester survey were asked to choose the most likely explanation for why certain celebrities were so successful. Their options included luck, innate talent, hard work, and even the possibility that the entertainment industry simply decided to turn certain people into stars. More teenagers chose "hard work" than all the other options combined.

The way Amy saw it, the most important thing right now was

to save almost every single dollar she made at her place of employment, a Subway sandwich shop. Toward the end of my visit she disappeared into her bedroom and reemerged with four business envelopes stuffed with crinkled $5, $10, and $20 bills. The first envelope, labeled "For Now," contained pocket money; the second, labeled "Just in Case," contained emergency money for repairs on her car or other last-minute necessities; the third, labeled "Never Touch," was a kind of pension or retirement account that she had vowed not to use until the age of thirty-five; and the fourth and largest envelope, labeled "New York City," contained her savings for the upcoming trip to Manhattan, in mid-July. This would be a pivotal trip for Amy, and if all went well, by then she would be well on her way to being remembered.

Mobs of Fame-Starved Children

AS MUCH AS I WANTED to accompany Amy Lumber and the others to New York City, the IMTA wouldn't agree to it. They have a strict policy banning members of the press and other outside observers. Yet as luck would have it, I soon met an agent named Cal Merlander who solved my problem. Merlander owns and runs an agency called Glamour Talent, which represents a number of mid-level television actors. Merlander is always looking for talented young actors, and one of the many places he likes to look is at the IMTA convention in Los Angeles. When I mentioned my interest in the IMTA to Merlander, he quickly assured me that he could get me in, though he didn't specify how. Several weeks later I met him at the Westin Bonaventure Hotel in downtown L.A., where the convention was being held. Cool as could be, Merlander sauntered up to the registration desk and slipped his arm around Jill Marlin, who was organizing the convention. Ever so gently he began to massage her shoulders. Moments later he presented me with a yellow ID badge identifying me as an agent who worked for him. "Stick with me," he said.

Merlander had a conventionally handsome face with deep-blue eyes and flat, symmetrical features. His skin looked freshly bronzed, as if he had just come back from a day at the beach. His hair was disheveled, but just slightly so, as if he had combed it and then roughed it up. All this gave him the appearance of the host of a game show for college-age singles.

Jill Marlin escorted us back out into the center of the lobby, where the convention was in full swing. The place was swarming with hundreds of contestants—mostly girls aged five to sixteen, dressed in strikingly adult fashion: miniskirts, butt-hugging shorts, low-cut camisoles, string-bikini tops, high heels, heavy makeup, and jewelry galore. Many of them looked as if they could be featured on the cover of a kids' edition of *Maxim* or *Playboy,* if there were such a thing. Most of the contestants were strutting around the lobby counterclockwise, following one another like lemmings in an endless migration that went absolutely nowhere. As dressed up as they all were, their skimpy fashions were actually quite uniform, making them essentially indistinguishable in the crowd. The most reliable way to identify individual kids was by the badges they wore, each of which contained a four-digit number. When an agent wanted to call over a certain kid, he or she merely yelled, "Hey, 4137, could you come over here?" or "Excuse me, 1249, could I have a word with you?"

The driving desire of each of the 1,200 kids in attendance was to launch a successful career in either acting or modeling. Accordingly, the convention includes several different events. Aspiring actors do "cold readings," recite monologues from memory, read soap-opera scripts alongside professional actors, and are videotaped doing TV commercials. Aspiring models participate in—among other things—a swimsuit competition, a jeans competition, and a makeup competition in which they have twenty minutes to apply their cosmetics before being judged. Most of these events are monitored by a gallery of scouts, agents, and managers looking for new talent. Indeed, the entire convention is predicated on the understanding that people like Cal Merlander will be there in the flesh, looking for the next Ashton Kutcher or Elijah Wood (both of whom are IMTA alumni). For this very reason IMTA officials kowtow to the agents, providing them with VIP lounges and serving them elaborate dinners, because they know full well it is the agents that these kids pay to see.

Jill Marlin led us briskly through the lobby and upstairs to a large ballroom where the jeans competition was taking place. We proceeded to an elevated stage at one end of the room. Directly in front of it was a roped-off section of seats occupied by roughly a dozen acting and modeling agents. Like Merlander, these agents were scouting for talent, but many of them were also judging the event for the IMTA. Several days later, at the end of the convention, the judges' scores would be tabulated, and awards would be given to the top contestants in several different age groups. Getting an award at the IMTA certainly doesn't guarantee success in Hollywood, but it is a good indicator that agents and managers may soon be calling. In this regard the convention functions somewhat like an *American Idol* competition, which may explain the IMTA's popularity.

"There is no question that *American Idol* is really helping the talent-convention industry," Merlander told me. "Kids are seeing unknowns, like Kelly Clarkson, become famous in the span of five weeks and then go on to win a Grammy. So it's no surprise that kids are so interested in these conventions. It's the same format. You perform on stage, you get judged, and you get a chance at being discovered. To these kids, I'm Paula Abdul."

In order to get into the roped-off section, Merlander and I had to elbow our way through a pack of cheering, camera-toting mothers, all waiting for their children to stroll across the stage in designer jeans. When this moment finally occurred, the mothers grabbed their cameras and alternated between cheering and clicking, cheering and clicking, cheering and clicking. One child, who was perhaps four or five, was so unnerved by this frenzy that he jumped off the stage into his mother's arms, as if to escape imminent danger. Finally a fire marshal asked the mothers to vacate the area because they were posing a safety hazard.

Merlander and I found seats and turned our attention toward the stage, where a procession of kindergarteners was walking down the runway and striking poses for the audience as loudspeakers behind us blasted techno music. I thought this scene was bizarre, but it wasn't nearly as disturbing as what I saw the following day, when a group of third- and fourth-graders dressed in padded bikini tops took part in the swimsuit competition.

The majority of contestants at the IMTA convention were children and teenagers, but there were also a handful of adults who, in between events, shuffled morosely down the hotel's corridors. Stephanie Howell was one of them. "This place is a joke," she told me bitterly when we met later in the week. "I can't wait to go home." Stephanie was a twenty-four-year-old nurse from New Haven, Connecticut, who had come here with the dream of becoming a soap-opera star. Things weren't going well. "You start talking to the agents and you get cut off by other people—mostly mothers coming up with their little kids," she said.

The agents, by their own admission, were much more interested in kids. The way they see it, Hollywood is overpopulated with adult actors—many of whom already have dozens of screen credits to their name—so why take on an untrained twentysomething actress with no track record? For the agents, the IMTA was a place to find kids who could be trained and groomed from an early age. As a result, the events featuring younger kids were the most heavily attended.

"This is a great place to see the whole country," Merlander remarked as we watched the jeans competition. "This is a Wal-Mart of talent. You've got kids of all kinds: fat, chubby, cute, small features, good teeth—you name it, it's here." To me, however, the convention seemed more like an auction, in which the kids were being scrutinized and evaluated with almost scientific precision. The kids themselves seemed to sense this, and many were only too eager to announce their height, weight, waistline, age, and ethnic origin as a sort of pedigree. One girl told me earnestly, "I am five percent French, five percent Dutch, five percent German, five percent Iroquois, ten percent Italian, five percent Irish, ten percent English, and fifty percent Mexican."

According to Merlander, a lot of Hollywood's big-name agents pooh-pooh talent shows like this one, but he maintains that this is one of the best places to discover child stars. "We found a kid named Aaron Drozen at a show like this, and within three months he was starring in a movie alongside Jim Carrey," he told me, never once taking his eyes off the stage. "When you talk about discovering stars, it happens right here. Of course, those stars don't like to admit that this is where they got their start, because they don't want to tell anyone that they paid five thousand dollars to walk across a stage a few times. They'd rather preserve the mystery of it all. And that's their right. But this is the genesis of it all."

An endless parade of children continued before us. A few of the youngest tried to smile bravely, but most of them looked completely terrified, even after the screaming mothers had left. The older kids, thirteen and up, tried to make eye contact with us, and as they did, they revealed a greater array of emotions. Some wore forced smiles. Others looked sad or even sullen. But the most common look was inquisitive, a searching glance, as if everyone wearing a yellow badge had something precious to give. Even a smile or a wink from one of us would do. Any measure of interest might suffice, as long as it provided a microscopic glimmer of validation.

"Do any of these kids interest you?" I asked Merlander.

"Not yet," he replied. "I'm looking for confidence and intelligence, and so far I haven't seen—" Quite abruptly Merlander snapped his fingers and pointed at the stage. "Look over there at 3058!" he whispered, indicating a girl of about ten who wore a Russian hat made of white fur. "Just look at the way she walks. She's so confident. I just wish she'd open her mouth so I could see her teeth."

"What about her do you like?"

"It's just a vibe," Merlander replied. "It's like the guy who found Lana Turner at Schwab's drugstore. He had a vibe—he felt it, just like we can feel it here. What you really want are the ones who love it up there. You want the ones who live for this. It has to be all about them. And they have to be intelligent. Basically, we want miniature adults. You want kids that look and act like adults and have little adult facial features and little adult mannerisms." For a rare moment Merlander took his eyes from the stage to look at me. He used his hands to frame my face and gradually pushed his palms together, as if he were squeezing me down to size. "If I could shrink you down," he said matter-of-factly, "I could make money with you."

"What about this girl?" I asked, pointing to an adorable four-foot blonde in pigtails.

"She's cute, but she's not superbright," Merlander said.

"How do you know that?"

"I just know—like this one over here," he said, gesturing toward a stocky girl of about ten. "I guarantee that she is from a town with a population of five thousand or less. It's obvious that she comes from a community where manners and posture are not that important. She's a farm kid. This one right here, 4702, she's a bright kid—the type who runs the parents. She'll be in the health care business. This one here is also bright, but in a more literary way. She'll be a writer. She'll be your competition in a few years. And this one here—she'll be a hooker."

"A hooker?"

"Yeah," said Merlander.

Eventually I asked him why he thought all these kids and parents had come here. He offered three reasons—or, more specifically, three types of families he encounters in this business. The first involves a precocious child who expresses an interest in becoming a star and then demands that his or her parents do everything they can to make it happen. The second involves a needy parent who seeks fame vicariously. This is the worst type, Merlander insisted, because the children are often miserable and the outcome is usually disastrous. The third type, which is the best in Merlander's view, can't be found at conventions like this. These were families that Merlander approaches randomly on the street or in a restaurant. "They're the best because they have low expectations," he explained, "and the kids have the support and love of the parents before any of this stuff happens."

"Would you send your kids to a convention like this one?" I asked.

"No, of course not!" he snapped. "This is just a fancy show. For my kids, I would call the agents directly. That's the way to do it. But these parents don't know that. The parents who come here heard an ad on the radio, thought their kids could become famous, and then sank five to ten thousand dollars into this on an impulse. These parents are not the analytical types. They're not engineers." Again Merlander turned briefly away from the stage and toward the hundreds of parents behind us. "Raise your hand if you are engineers!" he yelled. No one stirred. "You see," he said, turning back toward the stage. "The analytical types are not here."

After two hours of watching children strut around in their jeans, I needed a break. I decided to leave Merlander at the competition and take a quick stroll through the hotel lobby. I soon heard the sound of footsteps on my heels and then felt a tug at my elbow. "Excuse me, sir," said a young man of about twenty in a thick-as-molasses Kentucky drawl. "Would it be okay if I gave you my headshot?" Without thinking, I nodded, and he produced a large glossy photo with his name spelled out in block letters: BRENT GAVRELL.

"I'd like to be a celebrity," Brent said as we began talking. "To be honest with you, I'd like the whole deal. I see these celebrities on TV who don't like their picture getting taken, and I can't understand it. I want it all. I want the money, I want the women, I want the publicity, I want the people hounding me around trying to take my picture. I know that sounds really bad—it makes me sound conceited—but I guess in a sense I am."

Our conversation was cut short by a boy of about five who tugged on my other elbow and handed me his headshot. I took it. Suddenly three girls appeared, all pushing their headshots. I began to sense a rustling around me—the feeling one might get before being ambushed. In the next instant some two dozen children and teenagers were clamoring around me, urging me to accept their headshots. As I squirmed awkwardly, I was reminded of a time in Bombay when a mob of begging children surrounded me. Initially I felt only pity for those children; but after I had shelled out a few rupees, the mob tightened around me, and I became trapped and panicky as they pulled at my clothing and clung to me with wild-eyed desperation.

"I'm so sorry, sir," Brent drawled. "But this is what happens whenever a yellow badge stops."

I nodded and announced to the group, "Kids, I'm not an agent! I'm just a writer."

None of the kids budged.

As politely as I could, I forced my way through the crowd and took refuge in the men's room, where I promptly removed the yellow badge and buried it in my coat pocket. As I later realized, I'd been caught in what I dubbed "Ambush Alley"—the worst place in the hotel to be seen wearing a yellow badge, because it was adjacent to the convention's VIP room for agents and managers. When kids weren't competing in the jeans or swimsuit competition, they often lay in wait here.

After I gathered my wits, I returned to Ambush Alley, my badge now hidden, and took a seat by the water fountain without anyone's glancing twice at me. Brent Gavrell was long gone, no doubt in search of other yellow badges, and I began chatting with some kids who were still waiting.

One of the first kids I met was a waif of a girl in her midteens named Marnie Groski, from Mentor, Ohio. As we talked about the convention and how she had made her way there, Marnie told me that her story was pretty atypical. "I have cystic fibrosis," she explained.

"That means all her body fluids are thicker than a normal person's," added her mother, Linda Groski, when she joined the conversation. "Marnie needs several medications a day to keep her going. It's not an easy life."

Marnie explained that her condition had attracted the attention of the Make a Wish Foundation, which tries to make dreams come true for sick and dying children. Marnie's dream was to become a fashion model. With the foundation's help, she went to New York City for a photo shoot with Katie Ford, the legendary modeling guru. After the photo shoot Ford told Marnie that her height—just over five feet—made her too short for modeling. She suggested that Marnie try acting instead.

Ford's suggestion was actually something of a cliché in the modeling world. One agent at the convention later told me, "A lot of the kids here who are trying to be actors basically weren't pretty enough or tall enough to be models, so someone along the way told them that they should be actors. But the thing is, *they can't act.*"

When I asked Marnie why she wanted to be an actress, she thought for a moment and then said, "I guess I would like to travel, get my picture taken, and meet lots of new people."

Shortly after meeting Marnie, I bumped into Robin Gauer, another teenage girl from Ohio, who was also hoping to become an actress. Her chances were clearly slim: as I soon saw, she had a severe facial tic that periodically made her snort violently. "I'd like to be famous," Robin said. "I don't have any younger siblings. Well, I actually have a few half-siblings, but they're not around, because they live with my dad and he doesn't want anything to do with me. In fact, I don't even really know where my dad lives, and I've only seen my half-siblings like once or twice. So it would be nice if there were kids who looked up to me."

Many of the kids I met at the convention seemed to believe their dreams of fame were attainable not only because their parents and acting teachers said so, but also because stars like Ashton Kutcher and Elijah Wood had been discovered here. I heard kids repeat this fact over and over again—which was no accident. The IMTA and its member schools, like Personal Best, use this information for all it's worth. Helen Rogers, who owned the IMTA from the mid-eighties to the early nineties, told me, "Elijah Wood was discovered when I owned the company back in the early nineties, and people are *still* riding his coattails." Nonetheless, the formula seemed to work, instilling the convention's contestants with just enough hope to keep them going. Some had actually come to believe that the convention would transform them, virtually overnight, into megastars. Eddie Powell, a twelve-year-old who introduced himself to me as "Number 9708," was one such kid.

Eddie was a slightly pudgy boy with blond hair, apple cheeks, big brown eyes, and an infectious grin. He came from Battle Mountain, Nevada, and for the past few months his parents had been driving him several hundred miles each weekend to attend an acting school in Las Vegas. After Eddie passed numerous "tests," the school's director gave him permission to go with a handful of other students to the IMTA convention in L.A. Now that Eddie was finally here, he was convinced that stardom was within his grasp.

"I was thinking that I could keep living in Battle Mountain and have a house in L.A. that I'd rent whenever I'm out here for movies or TV shows that I'm doing," he said nonchalantly as he discussed his future. When I asked what, exactly, he thought would happen to him in the coming months, he replied, "I've been imagining that they will choose me to do three different things: First I'll do a commercial, because that would be the easiest. Next I'll do a movie. And lastly I'll do a TV show, because obviously that would take the most time."

Like Marnie and Robin, Eddie had modest reasons for wanting to become a celebrity. "I'd like to be famous because at school I'm just a common person. The popular kids at school like to make fun of me. No, that's not the right word—what they like to do is torment me."

Eddie said the prospect of becoming famous was something he dreamed about almost every night. "The dream starts with me coming back to Battle Mountain from the IMTA convention in a limousine," he said. "And when I get to school, there are security guards holding all the kids back, and some of the girls are fainting. And as I am walking through, I see the popular kids in the background saying, 'Hey, this kid is cool.' Suddenly I can hang out with the popular kids, but when they are acting mean I can tell them to lighten up and *they actually listen!*"

During one of my many conversations with Robert Thompson, of Syracuse University, he described the vindication he felt when he heard from old high school acquaintances who had once snubbed him. "I will get e-mails from people who have seen me on TV. Occasionally they'll come from someone I knew in high school—someone who didn't go to the prom with me, or slighted me in some other way—and those are some of the most satisfying e-mails I get. In fact, one could argue that the desire to be famous is simply the desire to alleviate pain—the pain of being bullied, the pain of feeling like a nobody, the pain of not getting the dates you want, and the misery of being below the people who inflicted the pain on you."

In all likelihood many other famous Americans have also viewed fame—at least partly—as a way to fill the void or ease the pain of a shoddy childhood. Marilyn Monroe, who grew up without a father and spent much of her youth in foster homes, wrote in her unfinished autobiography, "I knew I belonged to the public and to the world, not because I was talented or even beautiful, but because I had never belonged to anyone or anything else."

Indeed, given the number of celebrities who claim to have overcome a troubled youth, one almost has to wonder whether it's a requirement of sorts. The list includes Gregory Peck, Audrey Hepburn, Billie Holiday, Mariah Carey, Halle Berry, Roman Polanski, Sean "P. Diddy" Combs, Jim Carrey, and countless others. The pain and awkwardness of adolescence was glaringly obvious in a great many of the kids at the IMTA convention as they talked about bullies, a lack of friends, distant siblings, absentee parents, shortages of money, acne, facial tics, cystic fibrosis, and any number of other things. But they seemed to fervently hope that becoming a celebrity would right these wrongs. Perhaps their hope came from the pages of *Teen People*. Perhaps it came from the promises of entrepreneurs like John Robert Powers who offered secret formulas whereby the "least pretty" could "become the most popular" and even "girls with buck teeth" could "become movie stars." Whatever the origins of this belief, it seemed ubiquitous.

All this reminded me of the myth that prospective immigrants spread about American streets being paved with gold. There seemed to be an equivalent myth accepted by many of the kids at IMTA that fame opened the doorway into a better, happier world, which they were now about to enter. There was a sense that even a brief visit to this perfect world would forever change the way that people treated them, thereby opening the way to a new life where estranged fathers and schoolyard bullies alike would see the error of their ways and, at long last, offer their friendship.

Another thing that struck me about many of the kids I met at the convention was their apparent sense of entitlement. Eddie Powell, for example, felt certain he would become a star. As it turns out, attitudes like this—in which adolescents seem to expect a certain level of fame and admiration in their lives—may be far more common now than in the past. Research psychologists believe that over the past several decades narcissism has been on the rise among our nation's youth. Perhaps the single most compelling piece of evidence to support this theory comes from a study conducted by Cassandra Newsom, of the Virginia Consortium Program in Clinical Psychology. Newsom analyzed results of a personality test known as the Minnesota Multiphasic Personality Inventory, or MMPI. She compared test results from teenagers in the early 1950s with those from teenagers in the late 1980s. One of the most striking differences between the two groups was in how they responded to item #58, which reads, "I am an important person." In the early 1950s only 12 percent of teenagers endorsed that statement; by the late 1980s that proportion had increased almost sevenfold, to roughly 80 percent.

Newsom devoted very little time to analyzing this particular piece of data. It was another academic, a research psychologist at San Diego State University named Jean Twenge, who first realized the enormous implications of Newsom's findings regarding item #58. Twenge speculated that an important shift had occurred, and that today's teenagers had a great deal more self-esteem than those of previous eras. To test her theory she conducted a study of her own in 2001. Twenge analyzed the results of two other personality tests—the Coopersmith Self-Esteem Inventory (SEI) and the Rosenberg Self-Esteem Scale (RSE)—over a period of several decades. Both tests attempt to measure self-esteem. The SEI examines how subjects manage in various social situations by asking them to rate the accuracy of statements such as "I'm popular with kids my own age" and "My teacher makes me feel I'm not good enough." The RSE asks subjects to rate the accuracy of statements that are more self-focused, such as "I feel that I have a number of good qualities" and "I wish I could have more respect for myself." Twenge showed that between 1968 and 1994, college students scored increasingly higher on the RSE, and between 1980 and 1993, children and teenagers scored increasingly higher on the SEI. Just as she had suspected, self-esteem appeared to have increased dramatically among young people in America.

In her book, *Generation Me* (2006), Twenge argues that this rise in self-esteem is the direct result of programs in our school systems, which have increasingly promoted the idea that kids need to feel good about themselves in order to reach their potential. During the 1970s and 1980s, she notes, the number of articles about self-esteem psychology and education journals doubled, and during the 1990s that number rose by another 50 percent or so. Eventually scores of children's books on self-esteem made their way into classrooms. According to Twenge, one classic in this genre is *The Loveables in the Kingdom of Self-Esteem* (1991). It begins: "I AM LOVEABLE. Hi, loveable friend! My name is Mona Monkey. I live in the Kingdom of Self-Esteem along with my friends the Loveable Team." A page or so later kids learn that they can enter the kingdom only if they "say these words three times with pride: *I'm loveable! I'm loveable! I'm loveable!*" Over time, Twenge says, our commitment to teaching self-esteem in the schools has been institutionalized in programs and entire curricula. One popular program, called Magic Circle, requires that one child a day be given a badge reading "I'm great." The other children take turns praising the "great" child, and their compliments are written up and given to the child to keep. The ritual comes to an end when the chosen child is asked to say something good about himself or herself to the group.

Twenge concludes that our efforts to boost self-esteem in the classroom have fueled an epidemic of self-importance and narcissism. She isn't the only one to make this claim. Lilian Katz, a professor of early childhood at the University of Illinois, makes a similar argument in an article for *American Educator*, the official publication of the American Federation of Teachers. Katz begins her article by relating the following story. She was visiting an elementary school in an affluent suburb when she came upon a teacher who was asking her students to fill out a booklet called "All About Me."

> The first page asked for basic information about the child's home and family. The second page was titled "What I like to eat"; the third was called "What I like to watch on TV"; the next was "What I want for a present," and another was "Where I want to go on vacation," and so forth. On each page, attention was directed toward the child's own inner gratifications. Each topic put the child in the role of consumer—of food, entertainment, gifts, and recreation. Not once was the child asked to assume the role of producer, investigator, initiator, explorer, experimenter, wonderer, or problem-solver. These booklets, like many others I have encountered around the country, never had pages with titles such as "What I want to know more about," or "What I am curious about," or ". . . want to explore . . . to find out . . . to solve . . . to figure out," or even "to make."

There is other evidence that narcissism is growing among young people. The psychologist Harrison Gough, for example, found that college students in the 1990s were far more likely than those in the 1960s to support narcissistic statements like "I have often met people who were supposed to be experts who were no better than I." Twenge has done a study on narcissism, too. In 2002 she and two other researchers analyzed the results from 3,445 people who had completed the Narcissism Personality Inventory (NPI). The NPI asks subjects to rate the accuracy of statements such as "I can live my life anyway I want to" and "If I ruled the world it would be a better place." Unfortunately, the NPI has been in use only since 1988, so Twenge and her colleagues were unable to compare their results with much earlier ones. They did find, however, that narcissism scores were significantly higher among people thirty-five or younger. This led Twenge to two conclusions: that younger people are probably more narcissistic, and that everyone born after 1970 has been thoroughly indoctrinated by the self-esteem curricula of the 1970s, 1980s, and 1990s. In *Generation Me,* Twenge theorizes that American schools are essentially "training an army of little narcissists instead of raising kids' self-esteem."

If, in fact, our school systems are inadvertently bolstering narcissism, aren't they also inadvertently encouraging kids to seek the accolades of fame? The *Diagnostic and Statistical Manual IV,* which defines all officially recognized mental disorders, including "narcissistic personality disorder," or NPD, says that a narcissist is someone who has, among other things, an excessive and insatiable need for admiration. According to Keith Campbell, a professor of psychology at the University of Georgia who studies narcissism, fame is deeply appealing to narcissists because it offers a seemingly inexhaustible reservoir of praise and flattery. Campbell says this is true both for those with full-blown NPD and for millions of other Americans who simply have narcissistic tendencies. He notes that the NPI, the standard measure of narcissism, asks subjects to rate the accuracy of many statements that relate directly to fame, such as "I want to amount to something in the eyes of the world," "I like to start new fads and fashion," "I really like to be the center of attention," and "I wish someone would someday write my biography." Campbell concludes that the pursuit of fame is an obvious and often inevitable path for narcissists. And this may be especially true in this day and age, when celebrity vacancies appear to be so plentiful.

The biggest problem with many self-esteem curricula, says Lilian Katz, is that adults find it difficult if not impossible "to maintain a constant flow of meaningless praise." After all, how many times can a teacher tell a kid that he or she is great before the compliment starts to lose its meaning? What's more, if and when kids grow dissatisfied with that "constant flow" from their parents and teachers—or if for some reason the praise stops—don't events like the IMTA that promise fame become all the more attractive?

Interestingly, extroversion is yet another trait that appears to be on the rise among young people in America. In yet another study Twenge analyzed data from roughly 17,000 college students who had taken the Eysenck Personality Questionnaire, or EPQ. The EPQ measures extroversion by asking subjects a number of questions like "Are you a talkative person?," "Do you like going out a lot?," and "Can you get a party going?" Twenge discovered that on average, college students in the 1990s scored higher than 83 percent of college students who answered the questionnaire in the 1960s.

These three personality traits—self-esteem, narcissism, and extroversion—are enormously helpful if not downright essential for anyone who wants to become famous. Not surprisingly, this may be especially true of narcissism. In the early 2000s S. Mark Young, who holds an endowed chair in sports and entertainment business at the University of Southern California, conducted a study in which he gave the NPI to roughly 200 celebrities of four kinds: actors, comedians, musicians, and reality-TV stars. Young collaborated with Drew Pinsky ("Dr. Drew"), the host of the nationally syndicated radio show *Loveline,* on KROQ in Los Angeles. Typically Pinsky has a celebrity guest on his show who helps him dispense advice to listeners on a range of subjects, including drugs, sex, and romance. At the end of each show, as part of this study, Pinsky asked his celebrity guests to fill out the NPI. Young and Pinsky found that the 200 celebrities who had appeared on *Loveline* scored far higher on the NPI than did a control group of 200 business school students. And they found no correlation between NPI scores and the number of years these celebrities had been working as entertainers; in short, narcissism did not appear to have increased over time. In fact, of the four kinds of celebrities who participated in the study, the reality-TV stars—whose careers are notoriously short—had the highest mean scores on the NPI. Young and Pinsky concluded that "individuals entering the entertainment industry may already possess narcissistic traits."

Of course, some narcissism experts argue that the legendary hubris of celebrities *does* grow over time. Robert Millman, a professor of psychiatry at Cornell Medical School, is one of them. For many years Millman served as the official "psychiatric adviser" for the Commissioner's Office of Major League Baseball. In addition to counseling the nation's most troubled pitchers and heavy hitters, he has counseled actors, CEOs, politicians, and foreign princes. His main job, as he explains it, is to help them cope with the trauma of being famous. After years of observation, Millman concluded that the situations his patients repeatedly encountered—in which they found themselves surrounded by adoring admirers—appeared to be stoking their narcissism. He calls this phenomenon "acquired situational narcissism," or ASN.

According to Millman, most people with ASN have high levels of narcissism before they ever become famous. Success and public acclaim merely exacerbate the situation. Often a celebrity's entourage is most to blame. To illustrate this point Millman likes to describe what he calls the "fingernail scenario." A famous actor goes out to dinner with a group of friends. At the table he says his fingernail has been hurting him so much that he recently visited his orthopedist. This prompts someone there to say, "Most of you probably don't know this, but I recently underwent quadruple-bypass surgery." In response the actor asks a few questions about how his friend is doing and then goes right back to talking about his fingernail and how painful it is. In a "normal" situation someone might tell the actor to quit babbling, but because he is famous—and wealthy enough to pay for the dinner and perhaps even a limo ride home—it is quite possible that no one will say anything and the conversation will seamlessly revert to a discussion of fingernail injuries and the pain they cause. After several hundred nights like this, a person with ASN stops paying attention to the thoughts, feelings, and lives of those around him.

Though their views differ in many regards, Millman and Young clearly do agree that most celebrities appear to have high levels of innate narcissism. "It just makes sense," Millman told me. "In order to strive for greatness, on some level you really have to believe that you *are* great from the beginning."

Eventually Eddie Powell introduced me to his father, Wyatt, a wiry man with jet-black hair, a bushy mustache, and a severe limp. Eddie later explained, "My dad walks with a limp because of an accident he had when he was eighteen. He was digging a ditch with a backhoe on some loose gravel when the backhoe fell over and crushed his left leg." Despite his injury, Powell continued to work in the construction business, as was apparent from his heavy workman's coat adorned with the logo of a company that made sewer pumps.

Powell did not seem particularly comfortable at the convention—something he discussed quite candidly when we had a moment alone. "Up until now," he said, "my wife has been far more involved in Eddie's acting career than I have. In truth, she's been spending quite a bit of money, and that's why I'm here. I want to see where fifteen thousand dollars has gone in the past six months."

Powell was not the only one with reservations about the cost of the convention. Helen Rogers, the former owner of the IMTA, told me that she was generally dismayed by the direction the talent-convention industry had taken. Many modeling and acting schools serve mainly as "profit centers," she said, herding several hundred kids each year to various conventions like this one. "And everyone along the way is getting a cut," she added. "The school is making money, the photographer is making money, the people who print the headshots are making money. It's horrible. When you look at all the kids who have gone over the years, and when you consider the millions of dollars that have been spent, and you know that nothing has happened for them, you have to wonder whether there is a better way. But for many of these convention organizers and school directors, the kids are just numbers."

The numbers at the IMTA, Rogers adds, are impressive. After she sold the company, in the early 1990s, she stayed on as a consultant through 2000. During this time she kept careful records of the company's finances. According to Rogers, enrollment at the conventions in both New York and L.A. roughly doubled, and gross income more than tripled, between 1991 and 2000. The profit per contestant also rose dramatically. At the 1991 New York convention, for example, IMTA collected an average of $699 from contestants; by 2000 that figure was up to $1,308. (This includes what parents or other guests of the contestant paid to attend.) By the time she left, Rogers estimates, the IMTA was grossing more than $5 million annually for the two conventions.

Sean Patterson, an agent at the prestigious Wilhelmina Models, echoes Rogers's concerns. In 1996 a number of agents at Wilhelmina collaborated to publish a book titled *The Wilhelmina Guide to Modeling,* which has since become a classic in the industry. In a section of the book called "Model Beware," Patterson offers this assessment of the talent-convention industry:

> The people who run these hotel conventions charge registration and attendance fees anywhere from $300 to $1,500 to young guys and girls who want to be models. And what they do is, they invite one agent from this agency and one agent from that agency, and they offer these agents an all-expenses-paid trip to the host city—give them a stipend of $150–$200 for the day. It's a free trip for these agents. Now the advertisements go up—ads luring aspiring models by saying that there will be in attendance agents from Wilhelmina, Elite, Ford—European agencies too. So these young people, mostly girls, pay these fees to the conventioneers, who clean up. And there is usually no process of preselection. Anybody, regardless of ability or potential, can attend, if they pay the fee.

Tom Rowan, a lawyer at the Federal Trade Commission, says that some talent schools and conventions pose a "persistent problem." Some of them are outright scams, he says. According to him, some of the companies that run these schools or conventions may be charged with unlawful deception for, among other things, claiming to be selective when they are not, and telling consumers that they have "the look" and are likely to obtain work when that is not the case. "The problem is that it's not always cut-and-dried," Rowan told me. "Sometimes you can get into this gray area where it's not exactly clear whether an organization has broken the law — and there are probably companies that are carefully pushing the limits." Another problem is that "the look" agents want is often highly subjective and variable. Some agents at the IMTA told me that they were looking not only for "beautiful" teenagers but also for "pudgy" or "geeky-looking" teenagers, for certain specific roles. Thus, theoretically, a whole range of people have "the look."

Wyatt Powell seemed to have few if any illusions about how the IMTA operates. "I realize that eighty percent of the kids who are here probably shouldn't even be here," he told me. "I know that. Hey, if you're running a talent agency, you can't stay in business if you turn too many people away. So I look at this mainly as a part of Eddie's education. If this helps him become a better public speaker and feel more comfortable getting up and talking in front of people, then it might be worth it. But I'm still worried. Eddie thought he would come in here, get spotted, and become a star just like that. We need a safety net of some kind, in case things don't work out, and I'm just not sure where to find it."

That evening I met Eddie and his father at a sports bar on the fourth floor of the hotel. Over dinner Eddie told me that most of the kids at school, and even some of the teachers, thought "something big" was going to happen for him at the convention. Apparently his mother had arranged for an announcement to be made over the loudspeaker at his school, heralding his imminent success. According to Eddie, the announcement said, "We have a new star on our hands. Eddie Powell got the head part at the IMTA convention in Los Angeles, and he is going to be a model."

"There's a little pressure for you," Powell grumbled.

"I didn't know she was going to do that," Eddie said. "But afterward the kids started cheering. I was like, *I can't believe that my mother did this.* But it also felt pretty good. For the rest of the day everyone was asking me questions. Now the problem is they think it's pretty much a given that I'm gonna become famous—like it's automatic."

After dinner the three of us headed back downstairs toward Ambush Alley and the frenetic congestion of the hotel's main lobby. At one point, as Powell was limping along rather slowly, Eddie ran ahead. Powell turned to me and said, "I want to thank you."

"What for?" I asked.

"I'll tell you," he said. "Now, when Eddie comes home, even if nothing comes from this, at least he'll have something to talk about, because *you* paid attention to him."

"But I'm not an agent or a manager," I said.

"Yes, but you've got that yellow badge, and you can go into the VIP area, and you took an interest in him," Powell explained. "And that may well be the saving grace of this trip."

One evening later in the week I caught up with Cal Merlander in the hotel's main bar. We sat at a small table near the entrance. Most of the day's official events were over, but he was clearly still looking out for talent. He sat at the bar, eyes trained on the floor, eavesdropping on the banter of passing kids.

"Sometimes I'll just stand by the elevators for long periods of time and listen for voice quality and intelligence," he said. "Then, if I hear something promising, I open my eyes, and if the kid has the looks, I attack."

"Attack?"

"I can be charming," replied Merlander with a broad, toothy smile. "I charm the pants off the parents. Then I talk to the school directors who came with them, because if they get left out of the mix they can get irritable, so you have to kiss their asses a little too. That's the way it works. But you've got to be quick. I've got to get them before the vultures descend."

Rather suddenly, our conversation was interrupted by a young boy who had boldly walked into the bar area. "Excuse me," said the boy, who looked to be about ten years old. "Can I give you my headshot?" He had directed his question to Merlander who, unlike me, was still wearing his yellow badge.

"I'm not taking photos right now. But tell me, what's your name?"

"Joey," replied the boy.

"Joey, I saw you on stage today and you looked good."

The boy suppressed a look of skepticism.

"I'll keep my eye out for you," added Merlander.

Joey nodded politely, thanked us for our time, and then proceeded to the next table in the bar, where a raucous gang of agents was sharing a round of beers. "It takes balls to do what that kid is doing," Merlander said as he watched Joey give his spiel to the other agents. "I'd send my kids here just so they could learn to have balls like that. It's salesmanship really. They're a bit shy today, but by the last day here they'll be hungry."

Almost immediately another boy approached us. He introduced himself as P.J. and announced, "I heard you say some of the kids are shy today, and I wanted to prove you wrong!" Merlander politely declined. Next came a heavyset redheaded girl, whom Merlander also turned away. Gradually the bar was overrun with kids emboldened by the tactics of the others and clearly it was now only a matter of time before we would be swarmed.

"The reason this happens is that these acting schools actually tell the kids to spot the agents and introduce themselves," Merlander told me. "But mostly it's just the turds who do it." To illustrate his point, Merlander pointed at the redhead who had just approached us. "I'd bet your life that she isn't going to make it. But the truth of the matter is that you need volume to get the five percent whom you actually want to see. So the schools sell to the turds, and *they* finance it. It costs a lot of money to run this convention. That girl doesn't realize it, but she is paying money so that the top five percent can walk right over her. She's just a sacrificial lamb."

At this point the bar was crawling with kids, and since Merlander wasn't interested in meeting any of the "turds," I asked him to take off his badge so that we could at least finish our conversation in peace. "You didn't like wearing the yellow badge, did you?" he asked with a laugh. "You were so uncomfortable with it that you took it right off."

"You seem pretty comfortable with it on," I observed.

"I don't mind it," Merlander replied. "I like mingling with people—fucking with them a little. I love the attention. I enjoy people liking me and hanging on my every word. I guess when you wear this badge you get a little taste of what Tom Cruise feels like."

On my last day at the convention, I attended a seminar offered by Merlander, which took place in one of the hotel's ballrooms. The seminar focused on what parents needed to know before they moved out to Los Angeles with their children for "pilot season"—the 120 days between January 1 and April 30—when most of the casting is done for new television shows. The room was packed with parents, who were studiously taking notes as Merlander explained where they could rent a car, find an apartment, and hire a good acting coach. "You better bring a shovel," he'd warned me before the event, "because I'll be tossing out a lot of bullshit."

The seminar culminated with a speech that Merlander addressed specifically to the kids in the room. "Many of you are probably here because you saw Hilary Duff on TV and you want to be like her. Look, here is the deal. If you really want to do this—if it's painful to even think about not doing it—and it doesn't happen for you, I want you to remember: this doesn't mean that you are lousy. Okay? Got that? We might only see a quarter of the kids who are here, and that's the problem with these conventions. So if you don't get a callback, and fifty percent of you won't, you have two options: you can either go home and give up, or, if you really want it badly—*and you have to want it badly*—you can go home, learn some more, dominate your local market, and then come back."

The lecture got a hearty round of applause, and then Merlander was mobbed by parents. Amid the frenzy I bumped into Eddie and Wyatt Powell. When they learned that I knew Merlander, and was waiting to speak with him myself, Eddie asked if I would give him an introduction. Of course I wanted to help Eddie if I could, but I had serious misgivings about introducing him to a man who referred to so many children as "turds." But Eddie persisted, and reluctantly I agreed.

Eddie and I waited around until Merlander had spoken to almost all the lingering parents. Finally he turned his attention to us. "Who is this young man?" he asked with a smile. "I like him—he's got a great Charlie Brown look."

I introduced them, and Eddie smiled briefly before looking down at his feet.

"You want to be an actor?" Merlander asked.

"Yes, that would be nice," Eddie murmured. He seemed to realize that he was being evaluated, and this was making him quite visibly uncomfortable.

"Well, do you have a headshot?"

"Yes," Eddie said.

Merlander took the photograph, noted Eddie's badge number, and then shook his hand. "Tomorrow are callbacks. I'll see you then." Eddie flashed a triumphant smile, thanked us both, and then trotted away down a long carpeted hallway.

"He has a good kind of geeky look," Merlander said. "And I am looking for a chubby kid, because one of the shows needs them. But my honest opinion is that he might not be quite right for show business. He looked a little shy, a little intimidated, you know, he didn't look me in the eye."

I could see Eddie talking with his father far down the hallway, no doubt telling him the good news that he had just gotten himself a callback—and suddenly I felt a little sick about having played a role in giving him false hope.

"I did see one kid who I really liked today," Merlander continued. "He was reading his script when all of a sudden the fire alarm goes off. Everyone's looking around, and the kid doesn't stop reading. It was great. You see, that's what we're looking for. The kids have to be cocky. They have to look you in the eye and listen to you. And they may or may not respond. We don't want 'Yes, sir' and 'No, sir.' That's not going to sell. We are attracted to what ignores us, to what knows its value."

As we were walking back toward the lobby, we happened upon Merlander's budding star. His name was Ariel Barak, and he was short, with curly brown hair and dimpled cheeks. "Here's the guy I was talking about," Merlander said as he ruffled the boy's hair playfully. "Are you ready to get on TV and make some money?"

"Yes," the boy said casually. "I am."

Ariel Barak made quite an impression, not just on Cal Merlander, but also on a great many other agents and managers, who—in their capacity as judges—gave him high marks across the board. In fact, on the final day of the convention the IMTA gave him one of its highest overall awards: Best Pre-Teen Actor of the Year.

A few weeks later I arranged to meet Ariel on the patio of a coffee shop near the beach in Santa Monica. He was standing alone by an empty table, and he seemed remarkably comfortable among the adults sipping their cappuccinos and chai lattes. I introduced myself, and when I reminded him that we had met briefly at the IMTA convention, he replied dryly, "Are you stalking me?" There was a long silence. Then he smiled good-naturedly and laughed, but in a way that seemed both childish and adult. His rosy cheeks, still a few years away from needing a shave, made him look innocently boyish, as if he might burst into uncontrollable laughter if I told even a run-of-the-mill fart joke. But he also exuded self-confidence, as if he knew full well that—although he was just twelve years old—he was the one granting this interview and thus calling the shots.

"So," said Ariel. "What do you want to know?"

When I told him I was interested in hearing more about the fire alarm during his audition, he shook off a look of mild boredom, as if he was already tired of retelling this now famous bit of personal lore, and then nodded obligingly. "I was in this office, and a whole bunch of people were listening to the audition, when the alarm goes off," he said. "People started yelling and running out of the building, but I just figured that it was either a drill or someone would take care of it. I knew I wasn't going to die if I stayed in that room for five more minutes."

"You seem like a pretty confident kid," I said.

"Yeah. Because I don't doubt myself, and I never look down on myself—never. Most other kids doubt themselves. They think, *Oh, I don't look good,* or *Oh, I have bad teeth.* I guess that's why they do drugs. They get depressed."

At this point our conversation was interrupted by the arrival of Ariel's father, Zev Barak, who apologized for his tardiness and explained that he had been parking the car. "But you don't really need me," he added with a self-deprecating laugh. "I'm just the driver."

Barak was a slim, wiry man with close-cropped graying hair. He spoke in pithy, gruff sentences, which reinforced his air of austerity—an austerity that may have been forged by his stint as an officer in the Israeli army, where he worked as a commando behind enemy lines. Barak had moved from Israel to the United States with his three children and his wife, Merav, about three years earlier. They made the move because Merav had landed a fellowship at the Smithsonian, working as an archaeologist. Ever since then the family had been living in a quiet neighborhood of Fairfax, Virginia. "It's a very nice place to live," Barak said matter-of-factly. "People are not so tough. They say 'Hello' and 'Excuse me' when they pass you on the street."

Since coming to America, Barak had worked hard to set himself up as an importer of antiques—a career that was in its formative stages but had begun to pay off. Cash was still pretty tight for the family, which had made Barak reluctant to shell out the $8,000 for him and his son to attend the convention in Los Angeles. Ultimately a scout named Cecil Douglas had persuaded him to take the risk. Douglas had paid a visit to the John Robert Powers school where Ariel was taking acting lessons, and had sought out the boy's father soon afterward. "This scout told me that Ariel had the personality of five people," Barak recalled proudly. "So my wife and I decided, here we are in America, the land where the impossible dream comes true, so let's go for it."

In the weeks after the IMTA convention Barak and Ariel had moved out to L.A., rented a small apartment in Santa Monica, and begun keeping a busy schedule of auditions. Today, for example, Ariel had auditioned for a movie called *The Bench-warmers,* which would star David Spade and Rob Schneider. Tomorrow he would audition for a movie called *Yours, Mine & Ours,* to star Dennis Quaid. In fact, tomorrow promised to be especially busy, because it would also be Ariel's first day at Williams Middle School, where he had just enrolled.

"Are you nervous about starting a new school?" I asked.

"No," he replied. "My mind is like, *What the heck?*"

"He has been like this since he was little," Barak explained. "When he first got to the States, he was in a martial-arts competition, and the kids were so much bigger than he was. I was scared to death for him, but he didn't even bat an eye. That's the way he is with these auditions. It seems like he doesn't even care."

"I just go in there and do my thing," Ariel said.

"So, what will you do to make friends at your new school?" I asked.

"The same thing I did at my old school."

"When we moved from Israel, he had friends within the first week of school," Barak said. "And you know how at school there are always a few leaders? For like ten days he followed them around, and then they started to follow him around. I guess he just has something in his personality that people want to be around."

As the three of us finished our drinks, I asked Ariel if he ever missed his mother, who was back home in Fairfax. "Yeah, I guess," he replied coolly. "You know—can't live with her, can't live without her."

"And how have things been for your dad?"

"It is kind of hard for him, but I guess he's enjoying it. You know—no pain, no gain."

I asked Barak the same question. "In truth, it's very hard for me," he said. "I miss my neighborhood, my family, even my obnoxious dog. Basically, I try to shut my emotions down totally, and I become a soldier in duty of my son . . ."

Without missing a beat, Ariel jumped to his feet, pointed at his father, and yelled, "Drop down and give me twenty!"

Barak smiled uneasily, and then we all laughed, in large part because it seemed like the only way out of an awkward moment.

By the time our chat came to an end, I fully understood why Merlander—who was always on the lookout for "miniature adults"—was so interested in Ariel. He was good-looking, brash, energetic, and completely undaunted by the prospect of interacting with adults, let alone with kids his own age. He had not yet stepped foot in his new school, and already it was a foregone conclusion that he would fit right in. This turned out to be self-fulfilling prophecy. As I later learned, by the end of his first week at school Ariel had found a prospective girlfriend, made several friends, and gotten himself invited to a party.

In retrospect, it seemed obvious to me that this was the life Eddie Powell—and so many other kids at the IMTA convention—desperately wanted. The Westin Bonaventure Hotel had been overflowing with kids who were looking to escape their problems and find a new, more glamorous life. To me, it seemed both fitting and disappointing that the IMTA's grand winner was a kid who had apparently avoided even the standard adolescent pangs of awkwardness and self-loathing. More than anything else, though, what really seemed to separate Ariel Barak from Eddie Powell and all the other kids at IMTA was his sense of entitlement. Family members could make enormous sacrifices, agents could swoon, fire alarms could go off, journalists could come calling, and none of it seemed to faze him at all. Although he had not yet landed a big part, Ariel Barak was already a star in his own mind.

A Home for the Famous and the Almost Famous

JUST OUTSIDE HOLLYWOOD is a gated community named Oakwood Toluca Hills, whose welcome banner reads "Home to the famous and almost famous." Within the walls of this sprawling enclave one can find a furnished apartment, a rental-car agency, a general store, a dry cleaner, a beauty salon, a tennis shop, a car wash, and a busy schedule of weekly activities for kids, including a spirited karaoke session every Wednesday night. The complex was built in the early 1970s, and its many boxy buildings and orderly footpaths give it the look of a quickly constructed college campus. Still, Oakwood's facilities—including 1,151 apartment units—are in impeccable condition. Some of the communal spaces are downright luxurious.

Oakwood bills itself as the ultimate in one-stop shopping for actors—especially child actors—who need somewhere in Hollywood to stay until they are discovered. The list of celebrities who have passed through Oakwood over the years includes Hilary Swank, Jennifer Love Hewitt, Queen Latifah, Ricky Martin, Frankie Nunez, Aerosmith, and Jamie Foxx, just to name a few. The complete list, which is prominent on Oakwood's Web site, reinforces a general perception that this is *the* place to stay if you are moving to Hollywood and are serious about breaking into the entertainment business. Since the early 1990s the management at Oakwood has made a concerted effort to attract child actors by creating a special Web site (www.childactors.net), establishing a weekly schedule of events for kids, and inviting agents and managers for the "youth market" to come and speak on a regular basis. Oakwood courts these children and their parents, who are out-of-towners, primarily because they are willing and able to pay a premium to live in a family-oriented place with a national reputation as a steppingstone for budding stars. Not everyone who lives at Oakwood is connected to the entertainment industry. Many of Oakwood's units are inhabited by a combination of transient business people and long-term adult residents who simply enjoy living in a gated community. Yet the "showbiz kids," as they are known, are Oakwood's most visible customers—especially during pilot season, when the complex swarms with gangs of photogenic, stylishly dressed children. In fact, to stay at Oakwood during this time of year, one typically has to book at least nine months in advance—and should be prepared to pay around $3,500 a month for a furnished two-bedroom apartment with maid service.

Oakwood is just a few minutes' drive from the ABC, NBC, Universal, Disney, DreamWorks, and Warner Brothers studios. In fact, because the complex is built on steep hills, many of its balconies and windows look down on the valley below and into the legendary Warner Brothers lot. On clear nights, when the smog has thinned, children and their parents can peer through the darkness at the iconic "WB" water tower in the distance.

I first visited Oakwood in order to hear Cal Merlander lead a seminar on how to succeed as an actor in Hollywood. When I arrived, several dozen children had already packed into the residents' lounge in the North Club House, one of Oakwood's two community centers. Like the kids I'd met at the IMTA convention, they were mostly pretty young girls dressed in a strikingly adult fashion; but these girls seemed calmer, cooler, and more professional. Most of them had already attended a talent convention and gotten quite a few callbacks from managers and agents. These were the kids who had made it through at least one filter.

As we waited for Merlander to arrive, a woman named Rose Forti, whom the residents called simply "Rosie," made her way around the room saying hello to everyone. Merlander had described her to me as "the queen of Oakwood." Forti was a heavy-set, jolly woman whose jet-black hair had a Cruella DeVil–like white streak in the center. "I'm a very active person, and so I need a hairdo to complement that," she later told me. I would soon see just how active Forti was, as she hustled around Oakwood organizing hip-hop parties, Sunday brunches, and Valentine's Day dances. Much like the activities coordinator on a cruise ship, she was expected to make sure that everyone had a good time, and during her more than thirty years at Oakwood the kids had come to refer to her as "the Fun Lady."

When Cal Merlander arrived, he gave a rousing speech about what it takes to make it in the entertainment business. Then he invited the kids in the audience to practice their monologues, which seemed to be the real reason they were here: for an informal tryout of sorts in front of an agent who might give them advice or, better yet, offer to represent them. One at a time, the kids stood in front of the room and recited three-minute monologues while Merlander took notes. Afterward he invited them all to submit their headshots.

"I saw some good kids," Merlander told me after everyone had left. "But to tell you the truth, my main reason for coming here is to get in with Rosie Forti. My hope is that if a really good kid comes through here, Rosie will send them my way. So I'm just working it with Rosie—working it, and working it, and working it."

"How do you 'work it'?" I asked.

"I just tell her how great Oakwood is, and I tell her that she's the queen of Oakwood. Basically, I just give her props left and right. Rosie's a conduit for possibilities. I want to start coming here once a month to give these talks. There won't be a lot of return early on, but eventually, over the years, I'll get some action from the kids that she's going to send me."

Merlander and I paid a visit to Forti's office, which was wallpapered with photos of kids—much like the missing-children postings in post offices, except these photos were professionally lit, and all the children looked airbrushed to perfection. Merlander stared admiringly at several of the headshots and made small talk with Forti for a few minutes. I sensed that he was biding his time, laying the groundwork for his big pitch. Soon it came. "Rosie," he said offhandedly, "I just wanted to tell you that if you ever have a kid who needs an agent, you can have them call me."

"Can I?" Forti asked.

"Yes." Without missing a beat, he slipped his arm around her shoulders and announced with a smile, "Have them call me anytime."

I returned to Oakwood the following day for the weekly brunch. Each Sunday about two hundred residents—mainly "showbiz kids" and their mothers—descend on the North Club House for a morning of coffee, bagels, doughnuts, helium balloons, and general pandemonium. Gangs of impeccably dressed kids were squealing with laughter as they raced through the hallways. Not far behind them was Forti, carrying a basket of sweets. "If I keep feeding the kids sugar like this, I'll have to be calling security soon," she said with a laugh. Before I could reply, the Fun Lady was gone, chasing after another group of children.

That morning the North Club House reminded me of an upscale family resort. Children were playing tag, teenagers were swimming in a nearby pool, mothers were gossiping over lipstick-smudged mugs of coffee, and even a few grandmothers were knitting by the gas-burning fireplace. The adults were all women. In fact, throughout my entire time at Oakwood, I never met one father or husband. As I mingled with the mothers and grandmothers, a number of them said they felt as if they really were on holiday. During the week they spent long hours on the freeway driving their children to various auditions; but in their spare time they enjoyed the facility's luxuries. "A lot of mothers treat this place like a spa," an acting coach and longtime

Oakwood observer told me. "They exercise, lose weight, get a stylish haircut, and go back home to the Midwest with a new 'Hollywood' look." Makita Jones, a mother from Philadelphia, described her time at Oakwood as "the vacation of a lifetime." She went on to explain that she had taken a leave of absence from her job with Verizon in order to move to Oakwood with her son Darnell for a few months. "The cost is really more than we can handle," Jones said, "but we're taking it one day at a time."

A number of other mothers complained quietly to me about Oakwood's prices. "It can be hard," said Alexandra Getz, a mother from North Carolina. "So you find another family to room with, you eat a lot of mac and cheese, and you skimp on Christmas." Often the kids seemed to be aware of the financial strain their quests were creating. When I asked Getz's preteen daughter, Laurie, why she wanted to be famous, she replied, "So I can pay off all my parents' taxes."

As I strolled through the North Club House, doughnut in hand, both the kids and the parents I met seemed to be bursting with a sort of cabin fever, as if they'd been cooped up for weeks—and often they had. Many families at Oakwood shared apartments, living in close quarters and pooling their resources until they realized their dreams or packed up and went home.

Living arrangements at Oakwood could be extremely complicated. Some parents set up elaborate rotational systems whereby kids from multiple families would stay in a single apartment while the mothers took turns flying out to L.A. to watch over them for few weeks at a time. With some of the older teenagers the arrangements were even more unusual. I met a seventeen-year-old girl from Chicago named Gwen Sufi who lived with her best friend and a thirty-year-old nanny. The nanny was responsible for picking up groceries and driving Gwen and her friend to auditions. "It works out well," Gwen said. "It's almost like we have three sisters in the apartment." An aspiring magician in his late teens named Lucas Bentley, who was wearing a silk waistcoat and brandishing a deck of cards when I met him, had just moved in with an actress of the same age. The two were living on their own. "It is a little funny, because previously I went to an all-boys military prep school, and she went to an all-girls Catholic prep school," Lucas told me. "But I wasn't going to jump her just because she lives with me."

Such tight living arrangements seemed to compound the innate pressures at Oakwood. Like an elite New England boarding school, it attracts ambitious kids from around the country. "At Oakwood you are surrounded by people who want to be famous and book, and book, and book shows until they succeed," Lucas explained. "And unless this desire is in your blood, in your system, in your life, you shouldn't be here."

Tension was highest among kids of the same age, gender, and race, because they were inevitably auditioning for the same parts. The consensus was that an ideal Oakwood roommate or friend was someone who looked nothing like you; otherwise the constant competition would be unbearable. At the Sunday brunch I met two twelve-year-old girls from Dallas, Ali and Rebecca, who looked as if they could be twin sisters. The girls were not related but they did live together, and lately things had been tense because Ali was getting far more auditions. "I was going on, like, three auditions a week, and Ali was going on, like, two auditions a day," Rebecca lamented. When I asked her what she planned to do to remedy the situation, she remarked, rather optimistically, that she had just fired her agent. She was now with the same agency that represented Ali: Cal Merlander's Glamour Talent.

Not everyone I met that Sunday was brimming with ambition and nervous energy. Intermingled with the go-getters were plenty of glum-looking kids and adults who sat silently eating their free doughnuts, perhaps contemplating the prospect of yet another week in Hollywood with no auditions. Usually they were at a table by themselves, fidgeting with a cell phone or poring over some papers in a folder—as if the answer to all their problems had simply gotten misfiled. Some of these Oakwood tenants were adult actors. I met one woman from Texas, a petite blonde with a preternaturally taut face, who told me that she was putting her budding opera career on hold in order to break into the movies. (It wasn't working out.) Far more common among the adults, however, were mothers who had said good-bye to their husbands, given up their jobs, traveled thousands of miles, gone into debt, and had nothing to show for it but a thoroughly disillusioned child. One mother told me that she and her son had been at Oakwood for several weeks and had not yet had a single audition. "We've been sightseeing to fill our time," she said with a forced smile. "I hope it wasn't a terrible mistake to come here."

Even for the kids who were getting parts, a pressing danger loomed: growing up. None of them mentioned this to me explicitly, but most of them were operating on a rapidly ticking biological clock: they had to become famous before acne, stubble, and the general awkwardness of adolescence set in. This point was cogently made by Paul Petersen, a grandfatherly man in a dapper suit, whom I met toward the end of the brunch. Petersen had been an actor in his youth, and had seen the darker side of show business for himself. "I was one of the original sixteen Mouseketeers for Walt Disney, and I was the first to be fired," he admitted with a laugh. "I was a behavioral handful. I didn't realize that child actors weren't meant to be children."

Nowadays Petersen was the director of A Minor Consideration, a nonprofit organization dedicated to the welfare of child entertainers; his visit to Oakwood was part of an outreach effort to educate parents. "Most people in Oakwood are laboring under terrible misapprehensions about the reality of this business," he said. The greatest of these misapprehensions, he insisted, was the belief that child stars could become adult stars. By his estimate, this happened to only about one percent. "Parents just don't understand the timing factor," he told me. "Kids grow up, and it's impossible to gauge how this will change them—whether they will even be presentable—and usually it's doubtful that they'll pop out on the other side of adolescence and still be that marketable commodity they were when they were ten."

• • •

As far as I could tell, Oakwood's "showbiz kids" seemed to fit into one of three groups. The first was the most populous: first-timers, who had come to Hollywood with grand aspirations, and usually departed a few months later with a trunk full of bills and a newfound appreciation for home. The second was the rarest: stars, who had hit it big and typically left Oakwood with their families in a hurry to buy sprawling complexes of their own. The third consisted of families who'd been at Oakwood for years. The child actors in these veteran families were generally just breaking even—a billboard here, a commercial there, perhaps even a television pilot, but nothing that had catapulted them into the realm of conspicuous wealth or fame. And so they remained neither famous nor obscure, neither rich nor poor, stuck here in Hollywood's equivalent of purgatory.

During my time at Oakwood, I got to know several veteran families. Typically, they exuded a blasé sense of ease. They appeared to have seen it all over time—which they typically broke down into "seasons," short for "pilot seasons." The veteran mothers knew the basics of survival. They knew how to navigate the freeways around L.A., find the casting agencies, deal with the agents, and keep their kids on track with schoolwork. They knew not to rent a fully furnished apartment at Oakwood. Most of them had long ago moved a full set of housewares—sheets, pots, cutlery, plates, board games, TV, VCR, iron and ironing board—out to Los Angeles. And when they went home, if they ever went home, many of them packed their belongings into a cheap storage facility and kept them there until they returned. Above all, the veterans all knew one another, and they seemed to rely on one another for solace and companionship.

The most revered veterans at Oakwood were a group of two mothers and two grandmothers who had dubbed themselves "the Hollywood Knitwits." They met several evenings a week in the North Club House to knit and chat in front of the fireplace. I first encountered the Hollywood Knitwits on a Tuesday evening, after a hip-hop party that Rose Forti had organized. When the party was over, and the thumping beat of Usher and Snoop

Dogg had faded into the night, the Knitwits gathered at the fireplace. From a distance they looked like a Norman Rockwell painting. The resemblance quickly dissolved, however, when one of the grandmothers received a call on her cell phone from her grandson's agent. The other women rolled their eyes and kept on knitting.

I approached the group and introduced myself, and they did the same. The two mothers were a youthful-looking brunette named Alice Weymouth and a plump Mexican American woman from Dallas named Maria Lopez. The grandmothers were Ruth Huckle and Molly Boot, who went by the name of "Granny Boot." Ruth Huckle—a native of Phoenix, Arizona—had light-brown hair, a soft round face, and big gentle eyes. Granny Boot, which is what everyone, including her husband, called her, wore leather moccasins, pants cut off at the knee, and a flamboyant silk jacket with blue and green sequins. When I asked about her jacket, she replied in a thick southern drawl, "My husband owns a clothing store in Ozark, Alabama, where we live, and he couldn't sell these jackets for diggity-squat, so you know how it works in this business: what you can't sell you get for Christmas."

From the start it seemed clear that Granny Boot was the de facto leader of the Knitwits. She was both the most outspoken and the most skilled knitter, a fact that became apparent as the other members of the group periodically asked for her help. "Granny Boot fixes all our mistakes," said Alice, handing over a half-completed scarf. She went on to explain that this was their time to relax. Some mothers hit the exercise room religiously, some went to the salon, others surfed the Web. The Knitwits knitted. And while they were knitting, the women said, they made a point of *not* talking about why they were there.

"We all have our reasons for being here," Granny Boot said. "For me, it was about giving my thirteen-year-old granddaughter, Martha, a better home life." She paused for a moment, seeming to contemplate whether she really wanted to say any more. Then she shrugged and said, "One Saturday afternoon my youngest son, Ben, calls me up and says there's somebody he wants me to meet. So I go down to his restaurant, and there is this precious little child sitting at the bar, patting some menus. Her hands fluttered up to me, and oh, it was love at first sight. At that point they were still doing DNA testing to see who the father was, because apparently there had been a party, and it could have been any one of three men that night, but I told my son, 'I know this is *your* baby, because she looks just like me.'"

In the coming weeks and months Granny Boot did everything she could to bring her newfound granddaughter into the family, but this often proved difficult. When she took Martha to her church, for example, the minister refused to baptize the baby, because the parents weren't married. Indignant, Granny Boot stopped going to church. She also did her best to reach out to Martha's mother, Angela. Granny Boot hoped to mend the rift between Ben and Angela, but things took a turn for the worse when Scott—one of Granny Boot's other sons—came home and announced that *he* was interested in dating Angela.

"If I hadn't been sitting down," Granny Boot told me, "I would have fallen down. I said, 'Lord, have mercy!' I felt like this was pure white-trash behavior, but what could I do?"

"So what happened?" I asked.

"Oh, well, Scott and Angela ended up getting hitched," she replied nonchalantly, continuing to knit. She must have seen a look of surprise on my face, because she added, "You can go ahead and close your jaw now, because there is more."

According to Granny Boot, her granddaughter's saving grace was a small storefront in Ozark whose signboard read Hometown Model and Talent. "Believe it or not, as small as Ozark is, there was a talent agency. And Martha started going there after school." Eventually the kids from Hometown Model and Talent attended a talent showcase in Atlanta—a smaller version of the IMTA convention—where an agent from Hollywood approached Granny Boot and expressed an interest in representing Martha.

"I'm glad we came out here," she told me, "but it's been very costly for us. The thing is, I don't want her back in Ozark, where she feels pressure from a torn family life. Martha loves attention, but she doesn't get much at home. On Valentine's Day, do you know who sent her a card? Her grandma and her granddaddy did, but not her mama or her daddy. Now tell me: *How hard is it to write a note?*"

The other Knitwits nodded without looking up. They had clearly heard this story before, and the details seemed to wash over them like the lyrics of an overplayed song.

"Martha has made a good life for herself here," Granny Boot added. "This life is in her blood, it's what she wants to do, and if we can find a way to do it without going into debt, we will."

"Doesn't she have some auditions coming up?" Ruth Huckle asked.

"She has three tomorrow," replied Granny Boot. "And I am just really, really hoping that something happens, because we need that work in order to stay out here. We really do."

Not long after meeting the Knitwits, I found myself on a rolling, smog-shrouded Los Angeles freeway in the back seat of Ruth Huckle's green station wagon. I was traveling with Ruth and her ten-year-old grandson, Marvin, whom she was effectively raising as her own child. Huckle's son, Donald, had been in his early twenties when he fathered Marvin. "Donald was quite young at the time, and he asked me if I would help raise Marvin," she later told me. "At the time, I didn't exactly realize what he meant by 'help out.'"

Today Marvin had an audition for *The Benchwarmers,* a comedy about the world of Little League baseball—the same movie Ariel Barak had auditioned for a few weeks earlier. Apparently a cattle call had been issued for ten-year-old white boys, and now they were coming in droves to a small casting agency in Santa Monica, where they queued up to read lines from scripts that their agents had faxed them. A fax machine was a necessity at Oakwood, and across the complex, faxes constantly puttered in on curling sheets of paper containing the smudgy lines of scripts that had to be memorized on short notice. The scripts came as mechanically as clockwork, and the *Benchwarmers* script was merely the latest to sizzle across the wires and into the cramped one-bedroom apartment where Ruth and Marvin Huckle lived.

After the arrival of a script, kids at Oakwood often paid a visit to their acting coach for a dry run before the audition. Marvin occasionally went to an acting coach, who was currently teaching him how to cry on cue, but he saw no need to visit his coach prior to every audition. Instead he would borrow his grandmother's cell phone, dial his agent, and read his lines once for her — often from the back seat of their station wagon as they sped toward the audition. Today, after Marvin finished reading his lines to his agent, he switched off the cell phone and fixed me with a long, sober stare. He was a small boy with a raspy voice, freckles, big sleepy eyes, and a quavering wisp of a smile that at times seemed almost mournfully thin. "Everyone who meets Marvin says he seems like an old soul," his grandmother later told me. "Despite his age, it almost seems like he has been around for a long time."

As we drove westward on the freeway, Marvin and I discussed the benefits of being a child actor. "Thank goodness for my Coogan account," he said. A Coogan account is a protected bank account that all child actors are required to have under California law. "I love that account. Fifteen percent of all my pay goes into it, and no one can touch it, except for me when I am eighteen. The rest goes to my manager, agent, and my grandmother, so we can afford to stay out here. I don't really care about money now, but when I'm eighteen, I know I'll be obsessed with money."

"What makes you so sure?" I asked.

"*The Cosby Show,*" he replied confidently. "In every single episode Theo will say, 'Pops, I need some money!' And all the teenagers on the Nick at Night programs — like *Full House, Roseanne,* and *Fatherhood* — they always want money."

Our conversation was interrupted by Huckle, who declared

in frustration that she had taken the wrong exit off the freeway and had gotten us lost. "You need to go left here," Marvin said calmly. "This road will take you into Santa Monica."

"He has a wonderful sense of direction," Huckle said with a grandmotherly smile.

When we arrived at the casting agency, Marvin walked up to the front desk and filled out the sign-in sheet, which asked him to indicate his name, his agency, and which role he was trying out for—either the "jock" or the "nerd." Marvin circled "nerd" and quietly took a seat on a bench alongside several other skinny brown-haired boys of about his age and height.

As we waited for him to be called in, Huckle told me more about how she had come to recognize Marvin's abilities. "When he was little, Marvin had a bit of a lisp, so I took him to the University of Arizona to check it out before it got any worse. They told me that he was bright beyond his years." She decided to take him to the local chapter of Mensa, where he could presumably play with other child prodigies. But she discovered that Mensa's child division held gatherings only once a month. "This wasn't going to do it," she told me. "I needed something for Marvin to do more regularly."

After a little more searching, Huckle discovered a school called Big Time Kids that, like Personal Best in Buffalo, prepared kids to become professional actors. Marvin took to acting almost immediately, and when the school announced that it was offering a field trip to Hollywood, he and his grandmother signed up. During the trip the group from Big Time Kids visited Oakwood and attended a lecture by a well-known manager. "Marvin was a little chatterbox," Huckle recalled. "He was just seven years old, but he was taking notes and asking questions. You can't imagine it. So afterward this manager came up to me and said, 'I got to have this little guy.'" Not long after this Huckle and Marvin moved in at Oakwood.

Eventually Marvin was called in for today's audition. He briefly disappeared behind a closed door and then reemerged with a look of unflappable sobriety, as if this was just another day of work. Minutes later the three of us were back in the car, jolting to and fro in a snarl of rush-hour traffic.

Back at Oakwood, Marvin asked if he could run out and play with his friends before dinner. His grandmother agreed, and he flashed a rare look of boyish glee. Then he burst from the back seat of the car and sprinted down a small hill toward a knot of trees where some boys had gathered.

Huckle and I sat together for a while longer in her station wagon, and as we did, she told me more about the situation with Marvin's father. "We used to own a restaurant in Phoenix called Ringside Bar and Grille, and this is where my son, Donald, met his fiancée . . ." Huckle glanced around and then whispered the name "Cindy-Lou" so softly that I could barely hear her. "They never got married, but Cindy-Lou did get pregnant. She didn't feel that she could raise the child on her own, so Donald and I ended up with Marvin."

"But you're the one who's raising Marvin?"

"Yes," she said. "And it's been different than it was with my own kids, because with them, I was always so busy with Little League and all their activities. With Marvin, I can dote on him in a way that I couldn't with them. I also dote on him because he didn't have a mother. I almost try to make up for that—whether that's right or wrong, I'm not sure." Huckle stopped and sighed heavily. The car windows were rolled up tight, and the air had become hot and stuffy. Huckle seemed unfazed. She glanced out the window and then looked back at me. Her eyes were moist. "I can remember when Marvin was just three years old. I told Donald that Marvin was going to be on a billboard in Phoenix one day. And since then I have reminded Donald of the billboard thing. I told him, 'I've seen Marvin on commercials that played during the Super Bowl, so it is not unreasonable to think that I might see him on a billboard.'

"Sometimes I wonder whether Cindy-Lou has seen Marvin on any of those commercials. I wonder whether she would even recognize him. At this point I don't want his mother in his life, but I almost want her to see what Marvin has become. Almost like *Look at what you could have had!* I don't mean to throw it in her face or anything vindictive like that—I just want her to know."

When he wasn't going to auditions, Marvin Huckle—like many other kids at Oakwood—attended the San Fernando Valley Professional School, a nearby private school that caters almost exclusively to kids working in the entertainment industry. Each morning a little after eight a small caravan of cars would pull out of Oakwood and drive past a series of strip malls to a bunkerlike concrete building. From a distance the place looked like it might be a run-down storage depot. Inside were five cramped classrooms, only one of which had windows. The classrooms were connected by a hallway equipped with eight decrepit lockers and a cheap gray carpet. As threadbare as the school was, the teachers were quick to tell me that it was a step up from the previous facility, which had occupied a one-room storefront next to a tiki bar. Despite the new facility's improvements, the only real semblance of respectability came from a white wall showcasing framed graduation photographs of some of the school's alumni, including Janet Jackson; Tiffani Thiessen, of *Beverly Hills 90210;* Alfonso Ribeiro, of *The Fresh Prince of Bel-Air;* and Alexa Vega, of *Spy Kids* and numerous other movies.

My first visit to the school was midmorning on a Monday. The principal, a petite woman named Angie Peris, told me that she was a former accountant for Warner Brothers and had gotten tired of crunching numbers. "I wanted to get into education," she explained succinctly. "So I bought this school."

Peris invited me to observe some of the school's classes. The school secretary escorted me to a small room where a group of eighth-graders were—at least theoretically—just starting a class in U.S. history. As I opened the classroom door, a roar of adolescent banter ebbed into a hushed whisper. Two nanoseconds later I made the alarming discovery that no teacher was present.

"Are you a substitute?" asked a blond girl in the back row.

A rustle of excitement ran through the class, the sort that often precedes complete anarchy among kids.

"No," I said. I explained that I was a writer and was interested to hear about their experiences in Hollywood. The kids in the back row glanced at each other skeptically, as if they were considering a plea for clemency.

Finally a small boy with a feeble voice spoke up: "People back home think that this is really easy and that you can just come out here and get a job. Our friends don't realize how much rejection we get—waiting in lines at auditions and then not getting the part again and again."

"Yeah, everyone thinks it's the good life out here, with fame and fortune, when it really is not," another boy chimed in soberly. "Like the other day, I was talking with a friend from home on the phone, and he asked me, 'Are you in Hollywood or are you in the ghetto?' And I told him, 'Sometimes it is kind of the same thing.'"

For the next forty-five minutes or so the eighth-graders took turns lodging complaints about the disappointments of Hollywood, until finally the door swung open and a platinum-blond woman wearing sandals and a sarong walked in with a whimpering Shih Tzu in her arms. A collective groan resonated across the room. At long last the teacher had arrived.

At lunchtime several dozen kids poured into a makeshift cafeteria, really just a concrete patio fenced in by a row of imposing cast-iron bars. The kids chased one another around energetically, throwing elbows and occasionally stepping on the paws of the Shih Tzu, who barked and yelped as he scurried underfoot.

Amid the chaos I found Marvin Huckle having lunch with two friends—a pudgy, garrulous boy named Edward and a quiet blond boy named Clint, who was engrossed in *Common Sense: The Rights of Man and Other Essential Writings of Thomas Paine*. I sat down with them, and Marvin told me that today would be an easy day because he had no auditions. Edward said excitedly that he had just gotten an audition for a movie called *Whisper*. He would be trying out for the part of the devil's son. Clint mentioned vaguely that he'd long since retired from acting, and then mumbled something about how Thomas Paine was overdoing it with his demonization of the Loyalists.

I broached the subject of Hollywood again, and asked the boys to describe how they had imagined the place before they arrived.

"I thought it would be movie stars everywhere, and the gates to their houses would be open so you could look in and see them walking around their yards," Marvin said. "I thought people would be nicer and they wouldn't honk and give you the finger like they always do."

"I thought I would become famous, but I didn't know it would be this hard," Edward said.

When I asked where they had come up with their image of Hollywood, Edward answered quickly: *Entertainment Tonight.* I got the same answer from dozens of kids at the school. Many of them watched *Entertainment Tonight, Access Hollywood,* and *The Insider* religiously. These shows had both forged their impressions of Hollywood and continued to guide them once they were there. "This is how I figure out what's going on in the industry," another student named Johnnie French later told me. "This way I can, you know, fix the way I dress, the way I talk, and the way I compose music, according to what people want."

Since moving to Los Angeles, both Edward and Marvin had realized that shows like *Entertainment Tonight* tended to sugarcoat their portrayal of Hollywood, but this didn't seem to bother them. "I now know that these shows are planned out and fictional," Edward said. "Still, I watch them when I can."

"You ought to be careful, because they can be addictive," Clint cautioned, without looking up from his book. "You may wind up needing a therapist."

"Can you recommend a cheap one?" Edward asked.

Both boys laughed, and Clint carefully put *The Rights of Man* face down on his lap. "Everyone imagines Hollywood as the heart of stardom—the brightest and coolest place to be," he said. "And shows like *Entertainment Tonight* and *Access Holly-*

wood—well, they use this. Besides, people *want* to believe this is true, so they just close their eyes and believe. And like the other guys were saying, I think it's easier to get addicted to this stuff when you don't live in Hollywood, because then you're blind to the reality of life here, and you just believe what you see on TV."

Marvin and Edward had by now gotten pulled into a raucous game of tag, so Clint and I continued to chat. I asked him to explain why, at the age of eleven, he was already retired from acting. "I started acting when I was five and quit when I was eight," he said. "I did some music videos and a few commercials for little-kids' gear, but the stress to find work drove me to quit. Recently I've started acting again, but I've decided to work on a lighter basis. When I was younger, I always wanted to be famous, and I still think it would be nice, but I realize it wouldn't be some fantasy land."

"Why do you suppose most kids want to be famous?" I asked.

"I think people don't want to be lonely. They want companionship, and fame is a substitute for that, I guess. You know, if you are a star, you aren't lonely, because there are always paparazzi and people like that around. I think the motivation for most people is that they want to be loved. Because you have to figure—what is life like for most kids? If you live in a normal suburban neighborhood in Ohio, or some place like that, you go to school, you get hassled by the teachers, you come home, and you get hassled by your parents. And then you just stay in your room and watch TV and play video games all afternoon. Pretty lonely, isn't it?"

I asked him if he'd felt lonely after he quit acting.

"Yes, a little bit, I guess. It can be hard, because you get used to having everyone around you. You get hooked on the noise and the light. But I think that if you can't face yourself, then you shouldn't be doing this, and you probably need to sort some things out, because one day you won't have the job and the fame, and then—when you're all grown up—you'll really be afraid."

Clint paused for a moment, as if to mull over this final theory, and then added, "Well, I don't know for sure, because I have never been a grown-up."

The Rochester survey provides some compelling evidence that children who feel lonely, depressed, and underappreciated are more likely to seek fame, in the hope that it will make them happier or better liked. For example, teens who described themselves as often or always depressed were more likely than others to believe that becoming a celebrity would make them happier. Those who described themselves as feeling lonely were also more likely to believe that fame would have a positive impact on their lives—though the results were slightly different between boys and girls: lonely boys were more likely to say that fame would simply make them happy, whereas lonely girls were more likely to say it would make them better liked by kids at school.

Fame as a remedy for adolescent woes, real or perceived, may explain another of the survey's findings, in which African American kids were more eager for fame than their peers. When asked whether they would rather become famous, smarter, stronger, or more beautiful, 42 percent of African American kids opted for fame, whereas only 21 percent of white kids did. What's more, almost 44 percent of African American students said that their families would love them more if they became famous, while only 27 percent of white students said so. There are many ways to explain this data, but given the difficulties many African American children face—according to a 2005 article in the *New York Times*, two-thirds of black children are born out of wedlock and nearly half of those children who live in single-parent households are poor—it seems fair to suggest that hardship may be driving many African American kids to embrace fame as a solution to the problems.

Loneliness, lack of parental appreciation, and general hardship may be fueling many teenagers' desires to become famous, but another culprit may be television. Findings from the survey also suggest that teenagers who watch television frequently are more likely to believe that fame will improve their lives. For example, those who watch at least five hours of television a day are significantly more likely than those who watch just an hour or less to agree with the statement "Becoming a celebrity [will] make you happier." They are also twice as likely as those who watch an hour or less to believe that their families will love them more if they become celebrities. Of course, these statistics can be interpreted in two ways. The first is to deduce that the actual content of these TV shows is influencing how teenagers think and feel about fame. The second is to assume that kids who watch five hours of TV a day do so primarily because they don't play sports, belong to after-school clubs, or have many friends or attentive parents, and thus are lonely or isolated. If this latter scenario is true, perhaps it is loneliness, not TV, that makes these teens desire fame. In all likelihood, both factors are at play. A teenager may watch TV because he is bored or lonely, and then—as he sees more and more shows about the exciting lives of people in Hollywood—he becomes increasingly disillusioned with his own life and convinced that fame is an excellent way to gain recognition and appreciation from the world at large.

Some of the most compelling evidence about the relationship between loneliness and a desire for fame comes from question #20 on the Rochester survey: "If you suddenly became a celebrity—like a movie star or a rock star—what would be the best thing about being famous?" For a number of teens, the answer was simply companionship. "If I was to become famous, people would probably think I was sooo cool and they would all want to be my friend," wrote one participant. "A lot more people would notice me and my friends might want to be with me more," wrote another. "I would have a lot of friends and I would have a lot of really, really, really nice clothes," wrote a third.

Some clinicians believe that children who grow up feeling lonely or isolated are more likely to form addictions. Craig Nakken makes this case in his book *Addictive Personality:* "If you were raised in a family where closeness was not a reality, you are much more prone to form an addictive relationship for two reasons: first, you were taught to distance yourself from people, not connect with them; second, growing up in this type of family left you with a deep, lonely emptiness that you've wanted to have filled. Addiction offers the illusion of such fulfillment."

To be sure, none of the kids I met at Oakwood struck me as full-blown addicts—at least not according to the strict definition of the word. Their lives weren't being driven into the ground by cravings for fame. But that said, many parents did appear to be pushing their kids away from healthy value hierarchies. I met dozens of mothers at Oakwood who had taken their children away from friends, families, and schools in order to give them a shot at fame. Weren't these parents, consciously or unconsciously, encouraging their kids to re-order their value hierarchies by placing fame at the very top of the list? And in doing this, weren't they effectively pushing their kids down the path toward addiction? What's more, now that these kids had been deprived of their social networks, it seemed reasonable to assume that a void or a "deep, lonely emptiness" might soon form—the most obvious remedy for which, at least in the context of Oakwood and Hollywood, would be the validation promised by fame. Perhaps none of these kids were addicts yet, but the situation was worrisome, particularly for those who were neglected or needy to begin with. It might be only a matter of time before many of them were hooked—on both the instant rush and the deeper emotional validation that fame, or even glimmers of fame, offered.

If addictions really offer only the "illusions of fulfillment," as Craig Nakken puts it, then what fame seems to offer is the illusion of love. And isn't Hollywood, with its promise of glaring lights and endless attention, the obvious place to look for thunderous validation? Where else can one go to ostensibly be embraced by the whole world? This may at least partly explain why Sally Field, upon winning her second Oscar, stammered into the microphone, "I haven't had an orthodox career, and I've wanted more than anything to have your respect. The first time I didn't feel it, but this time I feel it, and I can't deny the fact that you like me. Right now, you like me!"

In the coming days I returned to the San Fernando Valley Professional School several times. On one of these occasions I had a quiet moment alone with the principal, Angie Peris. We talked for the better part of a class period, and I recapped parts of my conversation with Marvin and Clint. Rather suddenly Peris interrupted: "Clint told you that he was working as an actor again?"

I nodded.

"Poor Clint," she said with a shake of her head. "Clint's *not* working, but if this is what he said, I think we should just let him be. Clint is kind of a loner. He couldn't make it at a larger school. He has trouble with writing. His penmanship is almost illegible. He is mildly dyslexic. And he gets pushed from his grandmother to his mother to his father. He has three sets of textbooks, because we never know where he is going to be spending the night. And just so you know, as far as I can tell, Marvin is quite loved by his grandmother. The truth is—it's Clint who doesn't have that."

As it turns out, Clint's fib was actually small compared with the stories that many of his schoolmates told. I heard from teachers about a number of students who either told elaborate lies or embellished their lives and acting careers. In some ways, I suppose, these stories were no different from those that kids everywhere tell—tall tales about the girls they've kissed or the number of touchdowns they've scored—but these kids' stories, in classic Hollywood fashion, were often grand productions.

"We have a kid who was telling people that he had piloted a jet fighter, shot an AK-47, and had a pair of Michael Jackson's shoes," Raymond Garcia, an English teacher at the school, told me. The problem for Garcia and other teachers was that the difference between fantasy and reality was often difficult to discern. "The first year I worked here, this kid told me he couldn't do his homework because he had been in a parade," Garcia recalled. "I said, 'Yeah, right.' Then, the next day, I saw him in the paper." After this episode Garcia became far more hesitant to question students about their stories. "This is just part of the territory," he said. "As they get older, you never know if what they tell you is true or not. They'll tell you these outlandish stories about what they've been up to, and then—the next day—they'll bring in a picture of them and Puff Daddy.

"I don't know if all of this is really a bad thing," Garcia continued. "As an actor, you need to be able to invent backstories for your characters, and these kids are getting better and better at inventing outrageous realities." The most outrageous story he had heard in the past few weeks had come from Johnnie French, the fifteen-year-old who watched *Entertainment Tonight* and adjusted the way he dressed, talked, and performed accordingly. Apparently French had been telling his schoolmates that he was working for the CIA. "And some of the kids believe him," Garcia said. "Kids will think, 'That sounds like a cool fantasy—I'll usurp that and use it as part of my fantasy résumé.' And why shouldn't they? After all, this is Hollywood, a town where people aren't living in the real world anyway."

Toward the end of my stay at Oakwood, I attended the weekly karaoke night at the North Club House. This was perhaps the community's most popular gathering, and I was eager to see it for myself. The kids took turns stepping up to the karaoke machine and belting out the words to their favorite Usher or Beyoncé songs, briefly enjoying a glimmer of the limelight they sought. As they sang, their mothers bustled around pouring glasses of soda, filling bowls of pretzels, answering cell phones, and chatting about the events of the day.

I couldn't help noticing, once again, that I was the only man in the room. According to Chambers Stevens, an acting coach who had been working with Oakwood families for many years, this was no coincidence. "We have an epidemic of husbands who are assholes in this country," Stevens told me. "We're talking about men who haven't told their wives that they were pretty since they started dating. Fame or even a bit of attention through their kids serves as a substitute for these women and lets them feel that they are special."

As I meandered around the North Club House, munching on pretzels and talking to the moms, it seemed obvious to me that Oakwood was an escape from the unpleasantries and banality of life back home. For mothers coming from a humdrum existence in middle-class America, it was a reprieve from pushy bosses, sick relatives, and unappreciative husbands. But, of course, the reprieve was usually temporary. Few child actors at Oakwood found lucrative work. So the question became one that Wyatt Powell had posed to me weeks earlier: At what point do you face reality and pull the plug on your kid's dream of fame? Leaving the cloistered world of Oakwood was potentially very difficult, because as you drove down the hill past the giant welcome banner, you officially entered the ranks of those who had *almost* become famous. At this point it was finally time to go home and return to being whoever it was that you had once been.

I heard a number of stories at Oakwood about families or individuals who were loath to return home. For me, the most chilling of these involved Lila Hex, a mother from a small town in Georgia who had two daughters. One, Melinda, was paralyzed and lived in a wheelchair. The other, Isabelle, was healthy and said to be quite beautiful. Lila Hex had left Melinda with her husband and taken Isabelle out to Oakwood to pursue her dream of becoming a soap-opera star. Even though Isabelle never had much success, she and her mother refused to go home and return to their old life in Georgia. Chambers Stevens had been Isabelle's acting coach, and one day he received a call from Mr. Hex back in Georgia. "The father telephoned and asked me if I would help persuade his wife and daughter to go home," Stevens told me. "So I called Mrs. Hex and tried to persuade her that her husband needed her, and eventually she agreed." Isabelle, by then in her late teens, moved in with an actor she'd met. Meanwhile, Lila Hex set out for Georgia in her car, but apparently she had a heart attack along the way. According to Stevens, she ended up hospitalized somewhere in the Southwest, and her husband had to come and bring her home himself.

"The last I heard," Stevens told me, "Isabelle had moved out of Oakwood. She now works as a cashier at a grocery store somewhere in L.A."

Late in the evening, as the ruckus of karaoke night began to die down, I bumped into Granny Boot, who was getting ready for a night by the fire with the other Hollywood Knitwits. I told her that my time at Oakwood was essentially over, and with perfect southern grace she invited me to swing by the North Club House the following afternoon to say a proper good-bye.

When I showed up the next day, Granny Boot seemed to be in a reflective mood. I asked her how Martha's recent auditions had gone, and she told me that they were still waiting to hear from their agent. Then she shook her head and added that this might be her granddaughter's last season at Oakwood. "I have health issues," she explained tiredly. "I am a diabetic. And nobody in my family has lived to be seventy years old. That is something I have to look at." Even so, Granny Boot said, it would be hard to leave this place. "Acting has been good for Martha—certainly better than a shrink, anyhow—that's what I like to say. I used to perform at a theater back home in Ozark, and we did a dinner production of *Hotel Baltimore*. I played an over-the-hill whore, on the wrong side of fifty, who had some loose morals and liked to curse and booze. I can't remember her name, but she was a great ol' girl. Afterward one of the old Ozark society ladies came backstage and said to me, 'Oh, my dear, I don't know how you could say those words.' Like she never cursed in her life. I replied, 'Why, Miss Janine, you just look through the curtains, find someone you really don't like in the audience, and just hurl those words at them.' I guess with acting you get to become someone else for a while. Maybe that's what Martha is trying to do. Or maybe she just loves the attention. Whatever it is, she enjoys it."

But the problem Granny Boot could not surmount was

money. Martha simply wasn't making enough to cover her costs. During her four seasons at Oakwood she had landed some good work—including a major role in a made-for-TV movie—but it was never quite enough. "She made forty thousand dollars last year, which is the best she has ever done," Granny Boot said, "but the rent alone here at Oakwood is over thirty thousand, so we're not covering our costs. This has been a financial situation that involves sacrifice on a lot of people's parts. My husband is sixty-three, and he would like very much to retire. We're not wealthy people, and if we are going to stay out here, Martha is going to have to keep working. I told her that at the end of this year we'll look at the bank account, and if there is money we can stay, and otherwise we have to go home."

"What did she say?" I asked.

Granny Boot clasped her hands together and looked up at me with a tired smile. "Martha told me, 'Granny Boot, I will book a show, because I am *not going home.*'"

PART II

THE CELEBRITY ENTOURAGE

The Association of Celebrity Personal Assistants

THE WEB SITE for the Association of Celebrity Personal Assistants (ACPA) offers this brief and rather curious statement: "The evolution of stars and their personal secretaries has witnessed the emergence of modern-day personal assistants who are multi-tasking machines possessing the most resourceful, creative, insightful, and results-driven abilities."

Not surprisingly, the concept of personal assistants—or "courtiers," as they were once known—is an ancient one. In Roman times, senators hired "nomenclators," whose chief responsibility was to whisper the names of approaching dignitaries. Napoleon Bonaparte allegedly employed an assistant with the same size foot, whose primary job was to break in the emperor's new shoes. Some of China's Ming emperors maintained a court of 70,000 eunuchs. It only stands to reason that a city like Los Angeles, which is home to so many of the famous and the semi-famous, would have an organization for assistants.

When I first got in touch with Josef Csongei, the president of the ACPA, he was reluctant to talk with me because, as he sees it, celebrity personal assistants have not always been treated fairly by the press. According to him, this was especially true in the mid-1990s, during the O. J. Simpson trials, when O.J.'s side-kick, Kato Kaelin, was ridiculed in the media as a toady who did nothing but mooch off his boss. "That was a bad time for assistants," said Csongei, who slowly opened up to me. "Kato wasn't really an assistant, he was just a houseguest who occasionally ran errands for O.J., but not everyone realized that. So for a while people were calling us 'Katos.' We were perceived as, you know, hangers-on and freeloaders, because people did not understand the difference between being a groupie and being a hard-working aide. But the truth is that we work *very* hard. A good celebrity personal assistant is part agent, part accountant, part publicist, part cook, and, sometimes, part shrink."

Despite all the hard work and lack of appreciation that can come with this line of work, Csongei said, the jobs are still highly coveted. He noted that people regularly traveled great distances to attend a seminar titled "Becoming a Celebrity Personal Assistant," which was run by the Learning Annex and the ACPA. To prove his point he told me about Dean Johnson. In the coming weeks I heard this story from a number of assistants, including Dean himself, and every time it left me baffled.

The story begins one night in September of 1994, with Dean Johnson sitting at home by himself. Dean is a single, thirty-two-year-old business executive in charge of marketing and advertising at a sizable company in the health care industry. It is 11:00 P.M., and he is looking to unwind after a long day at work. The city where he lives—Columbia, South Carolina—is largely shut down for the night. Eventually Johnson notices a videotape that has been sitting on his VCR and collecting dust for the past three months. A friend from work gave it to him some time ago, and encouraged him to watch it. Now, with nothing better to do, Johnson pops the videotape into his VCR.

A talk-show set appears on the screen, the audience clapping enthusiastically as the camera zooms in on the show's host, Vicki Lawrence. Lawrence introduces her four guests, who are the celebrity personal assistants for Whoopi Goldberg, Roseanne Barr, Burt Reynolds, and Carol Burnett. As these assistants talk about flying on private jets and attending Hollywood parties, Johnson reaches for a pen and starts taking notes.

When the tape ends, it is midnight, which means it's only 9:00

P.M. in California. Without wasting another minute, Johnson picks up the phone, calls directory assistance in Los Angeles, and asks for the home phone numbers of the four assistants on the show. Only one of them is listed—Ron Holder, who works for Whoopi Goldberg. Johnson dials his number, and a minute later Holder picks up the phone. "He said I was very lucky to get through," Johnson told me. "Apparently, in the three months since he had appeared on that talk show, he had received about two hundred phone calls from people like me. He was in the process of disconnecting his phone, but he was nice enough to chat with me for a while." During their conversation Holder tells Johnson that he should consider attending the "Becoming a Celebrity Personal Assistant" seminar in Los Angeles.

A week later Johnson catches a flight to L.A. and attends the seminar. For three hours he listens raptly as a panel of celebrity personal assistants describe the details of their work: arranging for limo pickups, finding obscure pieces of expensive merchandise, making hotel reservations at the Four Seasons. In the last half hour the panelists take questions from the audience. Johnson recalled, "I stood up and my question was: 'I live in South Carolina. How am I going to do this?' And one of the assistants said, 'Friggin' move!'"

For someone like Johnson, with almost no connections in the industry, the notion of moving out to Los Angeles to become a celebrity personal assistant was beyond impulsive. He'd grown up on a small farm in rural South Carolina, where he spent much of his youth picking and selling tobacco. His parents were adamant that he get an education in order to ensure a better life for himself. Johnson went to college at Lander University, in Greenwood, and then on to graduate school at the University of South Carolina, where he earned an M.B.A. Eventually he found his job in health care, which provided a comfortable salary and a promising future.

"The irony of what I did is that M.B.A.'s are trained to be disciplined people who are rational in thought," Johnson told me. "There is nothing rational about leaving South Carolina and driving three thousand miles without a job—especially if you're giving up a good job in corporate America with a 401(k) and health benefits. You just don't give up that life and drive across the country to become an assistant."

The quintessentially American story of the guy in the remote hinterland who falls in love with the glamour of the silver screen, packs up all his possessions, and moves out to Hollywood to become a star is almost a century old. But Johnson's story offered a new paradigm: the guy from the remote hinterland who falls in love with the glamour of the silver screen, packs up all his possessions, and moves out to Hollywood to become an *assistant* to a star.

Of the thousands of people who work in Hollywood—agents, lawyers, stylists, publicists, business managers, and others—many gravitate toward the town's biggest stars. What is unique about celebrity personal assistants is that such proximity appears to be the only perk their profession offers. Most assistants describe the bulk of their work as drudgery—doing laundry, fetching groceries, paying bills. And unlike lawyers and agents, who rub shoulders with the stars *and* often make millions of dollars, assistants are not paid particularly well. According to a survey administered by the ACPA, celebrity personal assistants typically make about $56,000—not much money by Hollywood standards, especially given the around-the-clock obligations they often have. What's more, being a celebrity personal assistant is rarely a steppingstone to fame. According to the ACPA survey, celebrity personal assistants are, on average, about thirty-eight, right in the middle of their professional lives, and many if not most of the ones I met described their line of work as a lifelong profession. For them, being an assistant was not the means to an end but an end in itself.

Dean Johnson and I had our first conversation in the lobby of the Roosevelt Hotel. The hotel, which hosted the first Academy Awards, is something of a Hollywood landmark. When it was built, in 1927, the twelve-story structure sat among sprawling strawberry fields and offered a commanding view of a far more genteel Hollywood, where Model-Ts puttered up and down tree-lined lanes. Nowadays the view is bleak: Sunset Boulevard and its endless expanse of storefronts—an odd combination of seedy bars like the Viper Room (where the actor River Phoenix overdosed) and kitsch boutiques like Hollywood Hounds, where high-priced dogs can get "pawdicures," "bark mitzvahs," and "muttrimonies."

I found Johnson sitting on one of the lobby's many leather couches. He was a tall man in his late thirties, with reddish, sunscorched skin, green eyes, a shaved head, and a handsome Roman nose. He wore leather sandals, jeans, and a blue T-shirt with the words "Cooter's Tow Trucks." When he spoke, it was with a heavy southern drawl. One of the first things he told me after introducing himself was that he worked for Tiffani Thiessen, who gained fame in the 1990s for playing Valerie Malone on *Beverly Hills 90210.*

Before we met, I'd had no idea who Johnson's employer was. Nobody in the ACPA, Josef Csongei included, ever disclosed this kind of sensitive information about a fellow member. So I had a number of immediate questions, beginning with whether Tiffani Thiessen was even still regarded as a celebrity. As I later learned, the ACPA defines the term rather loosely, as "a person who is recognized nationally and or internationally within his or her field." Csongei was quick to admit that this vague definition occasionally makes things "tricky." "When assistants are applying to join the ACPA, we tell them to submit as many supporting documents as possible, in order to prove that their employer is in fact a celebrity," he told me. "We encourage them to send in articles from *Newsweek, Money* magazine, or even the *New England Journal of Medicine.*" Doctors, too, can qualify as celebrities, Csongei said—especially if they've won a great honor, such as the Nobel Prize. And according to the ACPA, there is no expiration date on celebrityhood. So yes, Tiffani Thiessen was indeed a celebrity, and Johnson was qualified to be an ACPA member.

"My thinking was kind of pie-in-the-sky when I first got

here," he told me. "I thought I would just work for Julia Roberts, or Jodie Foster, or Mel Gibson, right off the bat. I don't know what I was thinking." Instead he ended up working for Alan Thicke, who played the father on *Growing Pains.* Before he moved to L.A., Johnson had met a young woman named Gina Tolleson, who went on to become Miss World and the wife of Alan Thicke. With her help, Dean landed the job as Thicke's assistant.

"After watching that videotape about assistants, I just said to myself, 'Well, if they can do that, then so can I,'" Johnson told me. "And I guess I wanted to know, could I go from South Carolina to Hollywood and find my way into the life of a celebrity? I realized that would be a huge challenge, and for some reason I wanted it. I don't consider myself a vain person or a superficial person, but I would be wrong to say that we all don't like being close to something that's powerful, and entertainment is what captivates the world today. These celebrities are known around the world, and assistants are the gatekeepers. That's a powerful position to be in."

"So why not go to Washington, D.C.?" I asked.

"Most people can't even name the secretary of state, but they can tell you who Sandra Bullock is," he said. "It's sad but true. Most people would rather watch the Oscars than a State of the Union speech. And I figured if I was going to make a change, and go after something, I should do it the right way. I know that within the landscape of Hollywood, if you're an assistant, sometimes you might as well be washing the floors, but in Middle America they look on the profession with a certain amount of, well . . . awe."

After working for Thicke, Johnson had gone on to work for several other actors, including Noah Wyle, of *ER,* before joining Thiessen. In all these jobs he did his best to play the role of the genie in the lamp, accommodating whatever requests his bosses made.

"One person I worked for had to have their diet Snapples on the left-hand side of the refrigerator," he recalled. "It was a huge ordeal, and more than anything else in the household it had to be done correctly. It didn't matter whether the payroll came in, or the bills got paid, as long as the Snapples were on the left-hand side of the refrigerator. I don't make judgments, but I think celebrities generally have such little control over what the public thinks or what the critics say that when they get home, they need to exact monumental control. Often it's those little things that most of us don't even think about. The daily minutiae. Organic raisins versus sun-dried. And if you get organic raisins, they have to come from the booth on Third Street and not the one around the corner on Colorado Street."

The most trying moments for Johnson, without a doubt, were the tantrums. "I remember one time I was back in a dressing room," he said, "and I got such an ass-chewing from this celebrity over the timing of a publicity shoot. When I couldn't reschedule it, this person threw a tantrum. I couldn't remember the last time I'd been talked to like that, and I looked in the dressing-room mirror and I thought to myself, *What the fuck am I doing here?* And then, a moment later, I realized, *If the behavior is bad at this level, it will be worse at the next level, and you better just be glad this tantrum wasn't from a bigger star.*"

Despite all the bad behavior Johnson endured, he rarely if ever blamed his employers. If he blamed anyone, it was himself, and he did so both in conversations with me and in a self-published memoir, *Life. Be There at Ten 'Til: A Collection of Homegrown Wisdom.* There he writes, "I'm not placing responsibility on the admired. I'm placing responsibility on the admirers. We (I said we) set expectations. We hold people in regard without really knowing them. We assume that the personality reflected by celebrities during a talk show interview or during a performance is the actual person we should have over for a pot roast."

The way Johnson saw it, any angst he suffered over the "ass-chewing" he received was essentially his own fault, because he had made the mistake of drawing close to someone he should have simply admired from afar. To underscore this point, he invoked one of his favorite analogies, which involves the classic children's lullaby *Twinkle Twinkle Little Star.* "Like the stars we see at night, the radiance of celebrities is real," Dean told me. "And just like the song goes, we wonder *what* they are. But the truth is, often it's best to just keep wondering."

Johnson had apparently learned this lesson years before, back when he was a teenager in South Carolina. In one chapter of his book he reveals that he was an obese adolescent, known by his classmates as "Dean, Dean, the Butterbean . . . Fattest Man I've Ever Seen." Apparently his weight was so conspicuous that within days of starting junior high school, his best friend told Dean he was too embarrassed to be seen with him. Gym classes were the worst times for him. When his school instituted a policy requiring all students to wear gym uniforms, Dean hoped he would finally blend in. But the uniforms were color-coded by size: small was blue, medium was red, and large was green. Knowing he'd be the only kid in green, Dean forced himself into a red uniform, which was so tight that he could barely run down the court or pass a basketball. The next day he gave up and wore green.

"My defense strategy for getting through embarrassing and humiliating moments, especially at school, was to watch the clock and wait for the bell," he writes. "If someone was picking on me during a break, during recess or between classes, I knew a bell would eventually ring and a classroom setting would soon offer a safer haven. I realized that every moment had its beginning and ending and that nothing, whether good or bad, lasts forever." According to Johnson, this realization helped him cope with his celebrity employers years later. "A lot of celebrities are really high-maintenance," he told me. "They can be very overbearing with their barking, screaming, and yelling. But as soon as a tantrum is over, it's *over.*"

If young Dean Johnson was at one end of the social spectrum at his high school, Leigh Lewis, whom he describes in his memoir as a stunning beauty, was at the other. "She was a star athlete. She was a star student. She was a star. Period." His one and only interaction with Leigh occurred at the school's annual party, where yearbooks were distributed and signed. Dean immediately riffled through the pages of his until he found Leigh's picture, which he regarded with reverence. "I had never seen anything like it . . . ," he writes. "She was royalty."

Dean wanted to approach her but didn't know how to do it. "The little voice inside said, 'Keep your distance and don't go near the light. Appreciate her from afar as you would any work of art.' Instead, a bigger voice told my little voice to shut up and pipe down. Being a brave coward, I waited and made a weak attempt to compliment her as she was walking out the door." Leigh ignored this advance, and Dean was crushed. In hindsight he concluded, "Had I left her alone, my memory would still be of a stunning beauty unlike anyone I knew. Now, the memory was tarnished, and I wish I had listened to my inner voice. I would have been better off wondering. But I was responsible for my fantasy's undoing."

Johnson acknowledged that he'd learned then and there that it was best to admire such "stars" from afar—yet here he was, some twenty years later, working as a celebrity personal assistant. Even stranger was the fact that his employer was none other than *Beverly Hills 90210*'s Valerie Malone, once one of the most beautiful and exalted high school girls on TV.

During my time in Hollywood, I heard many other versions of this theory about getting too close to celebrities, including one from Ed Zwick, the director of *Glory, The Last Samurai,* and other blockbusters. Zwick has worked closely with stars such as Tom Cruise, Bruce Willis, and Denzel Washington. He had just finished working on *The Last Samurai* when I visited him, and his sun-drenched office in Santa Monica was littered with samurai swords that glinted in the afternoon light.

Zwick was a small, bearded man with intense dark eyes that darted back and forth as various assistants came and went, offering him faxes. "Look," he said as he shut the door to his office, "if you're going to ask me—Do I really believe that there is such a thing as a movie star?—the answer is yes. I knew a guy named Freddie Fields who was a famous agent. He created the agency that became ICM. He also produced *Glory*. Anyway, I remember the first time he saw the dailies of Denzel. Freddie was older than me, and he always called me 'kid.' And he said, 'Jesus, kid, look at him—he carries his own lights.' It is a wonderful expression, and there are certain people who are just lit from within.

"Of course, there are people I know who try to take from their proximity to these stars some amount of life force. There is a very strong heat that is given off by them, and it disturbs the air like a car engine on a cold day. And often, particularly when you're younger, you're drawn in by this. But curiously, these stars throw off very little heat. You can be brought into their light, and you feel the force of it, but inevitably that light is cast elsewhere, and suddenly you find yourself in a shadow. And it doesn't matter if you are a director or a personal trainer helping them with their abs, because it is the same heat. So there's a real connection, but it's brief and fleeting and finally not sustaining or nourishing in any way."

Interestingly, Zwick also held a countervailing belief that he couldn't allow himself to get too cynical or blasé about the allure of celebrities. This, he insisted, was one of the keys to being a successful director. "I have been out here in Hollywood for twenty-five years, and it's not as if my fascination with movie stars ever went away. It's not as if I've ever been able to fully divorce myself from being like a thirteen-year-old kid on line at a theater and looking at the movie poster. I hope I never do. Some amount of that feeling is important to have, because after all, that's what I'm selling."

For the past few years Dean Johnson has been a regular panelist for "Becoming a Celebrity Personal Assistant," the Learning Annex's popular seminar. The event is usually held at the Holiday Inn in Brentwood, a seventeen-story cylindrical tower that looks like the handle of a giant screwdriver rising out of the earth and looming over the city of Los Angeles. I decided to attend this event one evening to hear what Johnson had to say to people who were considering following in his footsteps.

The first person I met there was the seminar moderator, Rita Tateel, a curly-haired, plump, middle-aged woman wearing a bright-magenta cardigan. When she isn't teaching this class, Tateel spends her days persuading celebrities to attend corporate and charity events. "Most people don't realize that when a celebrity shows up at a big event, someone got them there," she told me. "My job is to help charities and businesses find the right celebrities for the right event or PR campaign. So if you wanted to get an African American celebrity golfer from the Midwest who is interested in cancer, I'd find him for you."

As the hotel conference room filled with roughly two dozen students, Tateel rose to her feet and announced that it was time to begin. She asked the students to introduce themselves. The first to do so was Clay, a well-dressed African American man in his midthirties who said he currently worked in the deli section of a Beverly Hills supermarket, where he'd had quite a bit of experience serving high-profile customers. "I believe I have what it takes to work in a celebrity environment," Clay said nervously. Next a middle-aged woman named Janice, who had worked in an office for thirty years, announced that she couldn't take another day of sitting behind a desk and answering phones. A heavyset woman named Samantha said she was an assistant to a family of makeup artists who had been working for Hollywood performers for four generations. "I love makeup, but now I'm looking to get directly into the celebrity world," she said. Last was Ingo, a fidgety, six-foot-tall Austrian with his hair tightly clasped in a ponytail. "I keep unusual hours," mumbled Ingo in a heavy German accent. Then he nodded emphatically, as if no more needed to be said.

Tateel thanked the students and then introduced the three panelists, who were sitting at a conference table at the front of the room. Tateel turned toward the first panelist, an attractive young woman who wore a nose ring, a camouflage V-neck T-shirt, and a black blazer. "Please welcome the personal assistant to a great artist, director, and actor whom you all know: Dennis Hopper. This is his assistant, Annie Brentwell." The classroom erupted with applause and several students began scribbling down notes feverishly. The second panelist was a blond woman with a deep tan, bright-red lipstick, and glossy pink fingernails and toenails. "Please let me also introduce the assistant to the queen of comedy, Phyllis Diller," said Tateel. "This is her assistant, Carla Kingston." After another round of applause Tateel introduced Dean Johnson.

Tateel began the three-hour seminar with a kind of drill-sergeant speech in which she laid down some hard truths. "First of all, you must be in good health at all times, because you are running a celebrity's life, and if you get sick their life can't just stop. So if you get recurrent colds, or the flu, or generally worn down by stress, this job is not for you. And you need to be flexible, able to work all kinds of hours, which means it's probably easier if you don't have a spouse, or kids, or pets, or even plants. This job often requires all your energy. And you have to be a can-do person. If there is one word that celebrities *don't* want to hear, that word is 'no.'"

The topic of saying yes and whether it was *ever* possible to say no came up often during the evening. Johnson offered this solution: "I tell my bosses right off the bat there are three things I *can't* do: I can't speak Spanish; I can't drive a stick shift; and I can't do anything illegal." Annie Brentwell had a different approach: if faced with an illegal request, she tried to find a compromise. "I've been asked to get drugs," she said. "And I've said, 'Okay, I can put you in touch with someone who can make this happen, but I won't do it personally.' This way I don't have to be a 'no person,' because I was taught to be a 'yes person,' and I think that's why I still find myself in this job."

Tateel interjected, "As a personal assistant, you could be asked to do anything, and you have to know your boundaries."

At this point Clay raised his hand. "Is it better to have a close bond with your celebrity employer, or is it better not to be close?" he asked.

"What you have to realize is that this isn't up to you," Brentwell replied immediately. "The bottom line is that you are *not* in control of the boundaries. So I allow myself to become whatever they want me to be. My approach is, you can call me whatever you like, and on positive days, if it's 'friend' or 'family member,' that's fine with me, but I don't think of them in those terms. And that's not to say that I don't have moments when I feel like they are my friend or family member—but I have to remind myself that they are *not*. That is the discipline that I have to keep."

Carla Kingston offered a more relaxed approach and suggested that she and her boss, Phyllis Diller, had become fast friends. "Mrs. Diller even put me in her will," she boasted. "My own mother never even left me much money, but Mrs. Diller was very generous."

Toward the end of the evening the discussion turned to the subject of perks. "Celebrities are always getting perks—first-class plane tickets and great meals—and you are like a second-hand beneficiary," Johnson said. "And it is nice to live a first-class life and to be picked up in the limo and have a thousand people screaming your name."

An awkward silence came over the classroom.

"Did you say a thousand people screaming *your* name?" Tateel asked.

"Not my name," Johnson stammered. "I meant, you know, your celebrity's name."

Tateel nodded and smiled.

"But there is a downside," Johnson continued. "When you're *not* with your celebrity, you go from being Dean Johnson who is assistant to a star—and who gets to fly first-class to South Africa—to just being Dean Johnson who has to fly coach back home to South Carolina. The other thing is, even when you are with your celebrity, no one really knows who *you* are. Often when you are on a movie set, people don't even know your name. You are known as so-and-so's assistant. You don't have a name. You're not a person—you're an assistant."

"That's brutal," murmured someone sitting behind me.

Weeks later, when I asked Johnson how he coped with the anonymity, he shrugged and replied, "That is a problem with this job—sometimes there is a loss of self." His admission struck me as both admirably honest and mildly disturbing. How, exactly, could one prevent this from happening? I recalled what Annie Brentwell had said about the mental "discipline" she maintained in order to remind herself who she really was.

Not long after the seminar I invited Brentwell to meet me for drinks at a hotel in Santa Monica. It was the first of several meetings we had.

Although she is in her midthirties, Brentwell has the looks of a rebellious schoolgirl, with her pierced nose, leather boots, black miniskirts, and camouflage shirts. I liked her almost instinctively, and I was often amused by her over-the-top warmth. She said things like, "Sweetheart, you know I absolutely adore you, but I can't possibly make it tonight." Yet underneath this veneer of cheerfulness was something very careful, almost rigid—especially when it came to discussing anything even remotely personal. On several occasions she told me, "I'm sorry, but as an assistant, I'm just not used to talking about myself."

At the Santa Monica hotel we sat on a patio by the beach and watched the sun sink into the dark chop of the Pacific. Almost immediately we started talking about Brentwell's job. "The mental discipline is incredibly important," she said as we sipped our iced tea. "For me, it's an ever-present attentiveness to the fact that you are just doing the job. You're not hanging out with your friend." The most important thing was not to express or even think about your own needs, she insisted. "If my employer has to think about me—even if they are not consciously doing so—it detracts from what they are doing. I don't have time for something to be about me. And neither do they. It's my job to take care of that person—to keep them feeling up—and that means being disciplined."

As far as I could tell, Brentwell's concept of discipline was not intended to keep her sane as much as to help her better serve her employer. She was constantly adjusting her psyche to become the perfect complement or counterbalance. She could play the humble servant, the trusted confidante, the cheerful admirer, or the supportive family member. And yet even when she emulated a friend or a family member, it wasn't exactly a realistic scenario because on principle, she was refusing to talk about herself or even to recognize her own emotions. The result was a pseudo-friendship, in which one person did all the talking and feeling, while the other deftly maneuvered to stay out of the way.

When I asked Brentwell how she took care of her own mental well-being, she laughed. Before working for Dennis Hopper she had worked for Sharon Stone—an even more demanding job. "This job can really burn you out," she said. "I imagine that psychologists wouldn't approve of what personal assistants do, because we're consciously choosing not to feel certain emotions when we are on the job. So we need sanctuaries. Wherever you can rest your head at night, even for a few hours, that is meditation and solace time. Even going to the bathroom can be a moment of private time."

As hard as her job was, Brentwell said, she hadn't found anything else that she liked as much. "After I worked for Sharon, I worked in an office as an assistant for a producer and then for a manager, but these jobs weren't nearly as satisfying for me. There wasn't a direct line to the person. I wanted more to do. Not just that, I wanted more of certain aspects of my bosses' lives." She got several different kinds of joy from being a personal assistant. The first, and rarest, came on those occasions when she could "play dress-up" and go to a gala with her employer. The most dramatic example of this was when she accompanied Sharon Stone to the premiere of one of her movies, and as a treat Stone allowed Brentwell to wear her jewelry and shoes. "Best of all, there's the limo ride and the whole experience of walking the red carpet, seeing the flashing lights, and having that very special feeling for one night."

Another, more common joy came on the days when Brentwell worked herself into a stupor. "If you have a demanding day, when you work from early in the morning into late at night, and you've done some important things and trivial things, too—like scooping up the dog poop or changing the cat litter—and you are dragging yourself back to your house at midnight, you just feel so good. In fact, you feel great, because you were able to do so much in one day. I get emotional even thinking about it. You feel like a superwoman. And on the days that they throw more at you, you almost feel better. I'm proud of my ability to lose myself and do whatever I have to do, even at the risk of health or sanity."

When I asked Brentwell what her friends and family had to say about this, she readily admitted that they worried about her. This turned out to be an understatement. With Brentwell's encouragement, I arranged to speak with both her parents. Her father, Ralph, a professor at a prominent business school, expressed serious concerns about his daughter's situation. "This is a very special world that she is in. Going to a movie premiere with Sharon Stone in a limo is a rush. But with Annie, I tell her that she can't be an assistant forever. It pays networking-wise, it may pay vicariously, and it may pay emotionally, but it doesn't actually pay." Ralph Brentwell also worried that his daughter was thirty-five years old, single, and so busy with work that she had no time to take a vacation, go to the gym, or even meet new people. "I've talked to her about this, and she hears me, but she has yet to act on it," he said.

What happens, I inquired, if she refuses to change her job or her lifestyle?

"That's when I get on a plane and go out there," he replied.

Linda Brentwell shared her ex-husband's concerns about their daughter's situation, but she placed much of the blame squarely on herself. A recovering alcoholic, she believes that her struggles with addiction took a heavy toll on her marriage and her relationship with her daughter. "Annie is a nurturer," she explained. "When I left the house, Annie's sister disowned me for a while, but Annie would fax me at work explaining what her dad was going through. She was 'Miss Fix It.' She wanted to make everybody happy—make everything right. She is a perfect made-to-order personal assistant, because she wants family and needs family. She would go out of her way to please whomever she is working for. She would go out of her way to bend her schedule to accommodate theirs, even without being asked, just the way you would do with a real family, out of wanting to please and make them happy and to get stroked by them. Really, the Hoppers have given her a great deal of freedom. And they would give her more, but she doesn't ask for it."

Annie Brentwell insisted that she was in the process of making a big change in her life. "Leaving this line of work is something I have to start thinking about," she told me. "I realize that I have to start weaning myself. Up until now it has only been about Dennis Hopper or Sharon Stone. But I have to remind myself: yes, there is Dennis Hopper, but there is also Annie Brentwell."

According to Brentwell, her decision to leave Sharon Stone was based mainly on the fact she "needed a break from the demanding lifestyle of 24/7 work." She wanted a job with fewer hours, which she ultimately found with Hopper. But she described her break with Stone as "excruciating." "It took a little over a year for me to get over it," she said. "I completely felt like I was failing by even having the thought of leaving."

Brentwell's use of the word "weaning" seemed telling. The *American Heritage Dictionary* defines "wean" as "To accustom (the young of a mammal) to take nourishment other than by suckling." It is quite plausible that a personal assistant—or someone in a similar position—might have to wean herself from the nourishment or validation she got from a powerful figure such as a celebrity. More notable than this, however, is the second definition: "To detach from that to which one is strongly habituated or devoted: *She weaned herself from cigarettes.*"

Many addiction specialists believe that we can become addicted not just to substances and activities but to powerful people as well. Craig Nakken, the author of *Addictive Personality,* suggests that one classic example of this is the kid who gets drawn into a gang and is willing to sacrifice his value system, his identity, and even his life to get close to the gang's all-powerful leader. Another is the college student who has a series of unhealthy sexual affairs with her professors. Ultimately, both can become addicted to the false sense of security these powerful people provide. The best example of this phenomenon, however, may be found in the world of cults.

Stephen Kent studies cults at the University of Alberta. He has examined how the Church of Scientology wooed Tom Cruise, John Travolta, and other celebrities to advance its cause. According to Kent, these celebrities are granted extraordinary privileges in the church. For example, he says, at a Scientology complex outside Los Angeles known as Gold, a gang of the church's "most committed members" were effectively brainwashed and pressed into "forced labor" to renovate Cruise's personal quarters. A former Scientologist named Andre Tabayoyon described the situation as being "equivalent to the use of slave labor for Tom Cruise's benefit."

Kent told me that celebrities fit quite nicely into the world of cults because they are already accustomed to living and working in environments where swarms of assistants and aides fuss and fawn over them. According to Kent, celebrities and cult leaders actually have a lot in common. He points out that most cult leaders have an "inner circle" that pampers them by laying out their clothes, preparing their food, driving them around, arranging their schedules, even handling their PR. "With both celebrities and cults the attendants feel a real sense of importance," Kent says. "They're helping the great ones to function. They're also so close to the power that they can almost see it and touch it—and that's got to be intoxicating."

There is a definite quid pro quo in these relationships: Followers get a sense of belonging, security, and importance; and leaders feed off their admiration and devotion. "You have got two sets of potentially unhealthy needs coming together here," says Kent. "The main problem is that those in the inner circle often pay a terrible price." After years or even decades of servitude they may finally leave, and when they do they are usually deeply upset by how much time has passed. Suddenly they realize they've lost family members, friends, and many chances in life. "Worst of all," Kent says, "they realize that their self-esteem or sense of belonging was built on a house of cards, and ultimately they were just serving the trivial needs of vain personalities."

Kent concluded that both cult leaders and celebrities run what he calls "greedy institutions" that exploit their followers. With celebrities the ramifications are enormous, because millions of us essentially belong to their cults. "Just think about it," he said to me. "We wear clothing decorated with their names, we buy all their products, we travel where they do, we talk about them incessantly, and the most we get is a slight buzz from being in their outermost orbits."

Admittedly, most of us engage in cultlike behavior from time to time when it comes to celebrities, but maybe what really distinguishes us is which orbit we are in. In the solar system of celebrity, if Annie Brentwell is on Mercury, perhaps the rest of us are on Pluto or even Neptune. And no matter which orbit we're in, to some degree we all appear to be warmed and held in sway by the same potent force.

Roughly once a month Annie Brentwell carves out a precious two hours to attend one of the ACPA's regular Wednesday-evening get-togethers. These meetings are typically held in the back room of a restaurant or a bar, where members can have a few drinks, unwind, and network. Brentwell first learned about the organization through Nicholas Cage's assistant, several years before I met her.

One evening, I attended one of these get-togethers at the House of Blues on Sunset Boulevard. Approximately two dozen assistants were gathered in a private area known as the Foundation Room Lounge, which was decorated with colorful tapestries, mahogany furniture, Persian carpets, and antique temple screens from India. At the door, Josef Csongei greeted the group's members as Rita Tateel handed out $1,200 worth of coupons for injections of a product she described as a new and improved version of Botox. "The idea behind this promotion is that if *you* use this product—and look good—then your celebrity will ask what you've done," Tateel told one assistant who was standing beside me.

Members were milling around the lounge, sipping drinks and catching up with one another. I introduced myself to a woman named Pattee Mac, who told me she was Nick Nolte's personal assistant. When I asked why she came to these meetings, she said that she enjoyed interacting with other seasoned veterans in her profession. They offered moral support without prying for details.

"This place is like a support group," added a young man named Gary Potter, who introduced himself as the former personal assistant to Dom DeLuise. "It is like the celebrity twelve-step program." Potter said that his professional relationship with DeLuise had just ended. "I was with Dom for three and a half years, but it was time to go. It's like any relationship. It's very personal. You know their lives and their private pains, and when you leave, it's like a breakup. It's sad. I'll miss the fun times we had together, but you just know when it is over." According to Potter, the key was to end things before you got too burned out in any one job.

Josef Csongei made the same point during one of our conversations. Csongei had once worked for the director and producer Stanley Kramer, whose films included *Inherit the Wind, Guess Who's Coming to Dinner?,* and *It's a Mad, Mad, Mad, Mad World.* "After working for Kramer, I needed something more low-key," he told me. "I wouldn't want an A-list job like Tom Cruise at this stage of my life. When you work for the big names, your own life can take a back seat without you knowing it, and you can become resentful. I was fortunate to recognize that before it was too late."

Many assistants used these weekly meetings to ask one another for advice. "As assistants, we get some very odd requests," explained Becky Pentland, who introduced herself as Roseanne

Barr's personal assistant. "Like when Roseanne wanted dancing poodles in tutus for her son's birthday. One of the members of the ACPA turned me on to a company that had a stable of circus acts. That's how I found the dancing poodles. And we also brought in this guy who lit his farts on fire, which was the hit of the parade." Pentland added that the ACPA was also an ideal forum for discussing "boundaries"—an especially tricky issue for her because she had married Barr's ex-husband Bill Pentland. Thus she was both Barr's assistant and the stepmother to her children. "When I'm working, I call her Roseanne, and when I'm not working, I call her another name, which I can't tell you. So it's like I try to be two different people. At work I try to be professional. I will say, 'Yes, ma'am, can I get you something?' And when I'm not, I'm more laid back, and shooting the shit. If she asks for a glass of water, I will say, 'F— you. Get it for yourself.'"

Midway through the meeting Csongei introduced a special guest speaker, a security expert named Mike Proctor, who had written the book *How to Stop a Stalker*. Some of the assistants listened with mild interest; others migrated toward the bar to continue schmoozing over another round of drinks. I spied Brentwell in the far corner of the room and went over to say hello. She greeted me with her typical exuberance, and we found a seat on one of the lounge's many plush couches. "I haven't been coming to these meetings as often as I'd like," she said. "But it's good to be here. Sometimes these meetings are like group therapy."

Brentwell told me that she had been feeling good about her job lately, because she expected to get a week's vacation in the summer—something she never would have gotten when she was working for Sharon Stone. Back then she couldn't even take a weekend off for a friend's wedding, because she was always "on call." Such events were all part of the personal life she had been forced to sacrifice. But now, at long last, her life seemed to be getting incrementally more independent. The very fact that she was here tonight, she insisted, was proof that she was serious about making more time for herself and her needs.

"People have always requested me, wanted me, even tried

to take me away from the person I was working for, and I feel proud that I was wanted like that," she told me. "But is this what I really want? Because there are other things I would like. I wish I traveled around the world more. And I do wish that I had kids, which I still want." Occasionally, thoughts like these made her consider quitting her job. But there was still time, she insisted.

One spring evening Dean Johnson invited me to his house for dinner and to watch the videotape of *The Vicki Lawrence Show* that had first brought him to L.A. The tape had been in storage for the past decade and he had not seen it since that fateful night in September of 1994. "It should be interesting," he said. "I'm kind of curious to rewatch it after all these years."

Johnson lived in a narrow townhouse on a sleepy back street of Studio City. His place was sparsely furnished with cream-colored wall-to-wall carpeting, two black cloth couches, and a glass coffee table strewn with a few copies of *Entertainment Weekly*. Johnson brought out a plate of cheese-covered bread from the kitchen. "Would you like some bruschetta?" he asked, taking special care to pronounce "bruschetta" with a hard "k." "That's the way I was trained to pronounce it when I worked as a bartender at Olive Garden."

With our bruschetta in hand, we sat on the living-room couch. For the next thirty minutes or so we watched a grainy copy of the now defunct *Vicki Lawrence Show,* until Johnson reached for the remote control and turned off the TV. "Looking back, it seems a little silly," he said with a sigh. "Part of me wonders, *What was I thinking?* The show seems cheesy. It's like watching an old rerun and thinking it's not quite as funny as I remembered it. And it makes me wonder where these assistants are now. As far as I know, none of them are still assistants. I guess . . ." He stopped himself and then began again. "I guess I'm not exactly sure what being a celebrity personal assistant prepares you for. Writers' assistants want to be writers. Assistant directors hope to become directors. If you have a recurring role on a UPN sitcom, you hope you'll get a recurring role in a prime-time series. But what does being a celebrity personal assistant do for you?"

He went on to explain that he was currently trying to break in to moviemaking. So far he'd had some encouraging success. His boss, Tiffani Thiessen, had helped him get financing for a short film called *Just Pray*, which he had written and she would direct. They were planning to start production by early summer. He hoped this might pave the way to a new, more creative professional life. But in the meantime he was still taking care of her dry cleaning and managing her groundskeepers. "Tiffani has been great to me," he said. "But she is the exception. In general, I suppose if you are a celebrity, you don't really want to give your personal assistant a job as an associate producer in your new show. Then you'd have to hire someone else to run your life—and they might not get everything just right."

When I asked how much longer he envisioned himself working as an assistant, Johnson hesitated. "There are times when I probably thought I'd be doing this forever," he replied. "But a sixty-five-year-old person can't be speed-racing across the city and down the freeway to get that special pink-elephant gift."

Eventually our conversation meandered back to the subject of his high school idol, Leigh Lewis. I asked if he had ever seen her again. He said he hadn't.

"I think she lives in Myrtle Beach now. She is married, and I hear that her family is beautiful. When I go back home and see a little blond family, I think of her. Or every once in a while I'll turn on the WNBA and think about how she used to play basketball. She was stunning in her uniform and her headband. I do think of her from time to time. I don't think about her in terms of that night with the yearbook. I don't think about her bitterly or morosely. In fact, looking back on that night with the yearbook, I think maybe she didn't hear me."

"Do you think Leigh Lewis had anything to do with your becoming an assistant?" I asked.

Johnson took his time answering this question, talking at length about all his various motivations for moving to Los Angeles—none of which had anything to do with Leigh Lewis, he insisted. Then, almost as an afterthought, he said, "Maybe I was testing myself. Maybe, on some level, I wanted to see if I could be close to something perfect without being so attached to it. But when I came out here, I didn't think about Leigh Lewis. I didn't see it as a rematch or a way to take on the crown again. And besides, there is a big difference between being fourteen and being thirty-two."

The Desire to Belong: Why Everyone Wants to Have Dinner with Paris Hilton and 50 Cent

RUSSELL TURIAK IS STILL, by his own choice and admission, one of the most loathed figures in the celebrity world. In his heyday he was a notoriously successful paparazzi photographer. Nowadays, however, Turiak is in semi-retirement, which means that he works only a few times a year, when the tabloid offers him a lucrative commission. At the age of sixty, he says, he is too old to be chasing celebrities around the country—this is a young man's game, he insists—and instead he now sees himself as the elder statesman of his profession.

When I visited him at his home, in Yonkers, New York, I was struck immediately by how fit he looked. When I mentioned this to him, he told me he was a martial-arts expert who was "still in crime-fighting shape." Then he thrust out his foot and swung it upward until it was level with his head. "Not bad, huh?" he asked, continuing to hold the pose. "I have said before—to do what I do, you have to be part psychologist, part detective, and part ninja." Eventually, when I made it clear that I was sufficiently impressed, Turiak broke his pose and took a bow.

At first glance he didn't look particularly tough. He had sharp green eyes and a fleshy, boyish face with a peachy complexion that appeared to have been touched up with makeup. This, combined with his well-coiffed black hair, gave him the vaguely generic good looks of a TV anchorman. For the most part he was congenial, but when it came to talking shop, a toughness surfaced, and he assumed the speech and manner of a mercenary or a big-game hunter—which was exactly how he saw himself. This became apparent as he regaled me with stories about tracking down and photographing Steve McQueen.

"It's all just a game," Turiak told me as we sat in his kitchen. "And my best game was against the ultimate game player, Steve McQueen, the king of cool. In *The Great Escape,* do you remember the scene where he jumped the fence on his motorcycle? Well, he did that stunt himself. And he did everything to keep me from getting pictures of him. But in the end I won. I beat him."

When I asked him to tell me more about what it took to be a topnotch paparazzo, he led me down a narrow hallway to a giant framed display of photographs of roughly thirty celebrities, including Mick Jagger, Mike Tyson, Tom Cruise, and Barbra Streisand—all with their tongues sticking out. "These are my tongue pictures," Turiak said. "Everyone inevitably sticks their tongue out—especially when they're trying to be careful with what they're saying. So they hesitate, and then it happens." He paused rather melodramatically and then he drew closer to make his point. "Doing what I do, you watch people. You become a behaviorist. It's like photographing wildlife. You become familiar with the nature of the animal you're photographing—and it's the same way with celebrities."

Turiak eventually led me down into the basement of his house, where he had his office—a large, dimly lit room with about thirty filing cabinets. The walls were hung with framed magazine covers from the *Star,* the *Globe,* and the *National Enquirer.* In the course of his career Turiak had shot roughly four hundred covers—almost all for tabloids, and almost all featuring a celebrity of one kind or another. But the covers represented only a small fraction of his photographs: tens of thousands of others, never published, were stowed away in these cabinets. Periodically he got calls from people who wanted to buy or use some of these photos. His entire Jacqueline Onassis collection, for example, was on loan to the History Channel for a documentary it was making.

"Everything is organized alphabetically," he told me. "So let's say you wanted to find the pictures of Steve McQueen I told you about—they would be over here . . ." He walked past several cabinets until he came to one labeled "M." He then heaved open a giant sliding drawer and began flipping through a series of dog-eared paper folders. Under his breath, he muttered softly as he perused his files: "Madonna . . . Madonna with Sean Penn . . . Madonna and Sean Penn in Hong Kong . . . I am looking for Mc— . . . Okay, here we go . . . John McEnroe . . . Steve McQueen . . . Steve McQueen with his wife Barbara Minty . . . Ah hah!" He pulled out the file and showed me several shots of Steve McQueen kissing his wife. There was nothing glamorous or sexy about them, they weren't even particularly good photographs—just grainy close-ups of a middle-aged man and his wife having a moment to themselves in a small boat on a lake in Illinois.

"Do you ever talk with any of the celebrities you photograph?" I asked.

"Sure," Turiak said. "Jack Nicholson once asked me, 'How many pictures do you have to take?' And I said, 'You know when you do a movie and you do take after take after take to get it right?' And he understood. I try to say something back that'll either make sense to them or make them crack a smile, so they'll say, 'He's a likable idiot,' or 'He's a likable asshole.' And I get along with a lot of them. Jack Nicholson and Sylvester Stallone have always been good to me. Michael Douglas always says hello to me."

Turiak gathered up the photographs and put them back in the filing cabinet. For the next half hour or so he told me stories as he searched through his files and pulled out various pictures. At one point, as we got to talking about the issue of privacy, he immediately grew defensive. "This is not about privacy," he said in a measured voice, as a twitch of anger rippled along the contours of his mouth. "This is about publicity and who gets to control it. These celebrities would kiss your ass in Macy's window on New Year's Eve to get publicity when they want it and need it, but once they have it, *they* want to control it. They're pimping themselves just like the rest of us—they're just doing it on a grander scale.

"When they go into show business, they enter into a deal with the devil. They know what the publicity is about and how the machine works: the more successful they become, the more they are going to be pursued. They know the media is out there. They go into the business accepting this, and then they become so rich and powerful, and so sought-after and so ass-kissed by all these agents and managers and publicists and lawyers and stand-ins and personal assistants, that they wouldn't know how to find their own ass if someone wasn't kissing it for them. But they've made a deal with the devil, and the way I see it, I am the devil's helper."

I nodded awkwardly.

Turiak took a deep sigh as if to gather himself, and a moment of silence passed.

"Would you like to see the rest of the house?" he asked in a strained but polite manner.

For the next half hour or so he paraded me through a series of cramped rooms filled with a hodgepodge of furniture, much of which looked to be from the 1970s. On the way back to the kitchen, as the tour neared its end, we passed the "tongue photos" and another, even larger framed display. I stopped for a moment to inspect this display, and I noticed that it contained three notes that Jacqueline Onassis had sent to Turiak in the early 1980s. The first one was three sentences long and it thanked him for sending photographs that he had taken of Caroline Kennedy at her graduation. The other two letters—which were almost identical in tone, format, and length—thanked him for sending photos of the Kennedy children on other occasions.

As I read these letters, Turiak stood behind me, looking over my shoulder. "Sometimes I send people copies of the photos I take of them," he said. "And several of them have sent me nice notes or have come over and thanked me. I have a really nice note from Donald Trump, a beautiful note from Oprah, a great note from Steve Allen, and these from Jacqueline Kennedy Onassis."

Turiak was particularly fond of the letter that Onassis had sent him in July of 1983 after John F. Kennedy Jr.'s graduation. The wording of this note was almost identical to that of the previous notes, with a few minor grammatical differences, including that at one point she used the pronoun "I." And instead of typing out "Dear Mr. Turiak," as she had done in the earlier letters, she wrote the phrase by hand. All this led Turiak to believe that Onassis had grown somewhat fonder of him over time. "You could see that the others sort of follow a tone of formality out of a book on how to write thank-you notes for people who are well-bred. But this last one is very personal," he said. "It's almost like she was really trying to tell me that it meant a great deal to her, and when I read this last note, it really touched me."

It did seem odd that Onassis and the other celebrities had written notes to a man who was essentially stalking them. Was this standard protocol for "well-bred" public figures? Or had they written out of self-interest, in the hope that if they treated Turiak as a human being, he would treat them as human beings? If so, their strategy seemed to have worked: Turiak was reverent toward those celebrities who had taken the time to write him back.

Despite his fury about how "ass-kissed" celebrities were, and his insistence that their contempt didn't faze him, Turiak clearly fancied the notion of himself as a pen pal of Oprah and Jackie O. He enjoyed playing some role in their lives. Even when he spoke of celebrities who had shunned him, like Steve McQueen, he seemed to assume that he and the celebrity were on some sort of equal footing—like age-old rivals who shared both hatred and grudging respect. This was true with Burt Reynolds, whom Turiak had once engaged in a fistfight. By playing the role of the camera-toting villain, he had become Reynolds's antagonist—and antagonists always play a crucial role in the narratives of protagonists.

Turiak clearly longed to be a part of the celebrity world, and at one time he had been. During the holiday season, for example, he usually traveled to Aspen to photograph celebrities skiing. In the early spring he went to California to cover the award shows. His encounters along the way, with Jack Nicholson or Sylvester Stallone, meant a great deal to him. He spoke with awe of a thirty-minute conversation he'd once had with Bob Dylan—whom he called "Zimmy"—on the pier in Santa Monica. And he spoke even more reverently of John Lennon. "He was probably the only person who made my knees shake when I talked to him," Turiak told me. "When he died, I was heartbroken. I cried. I really did."

Although Turiak sometimes gushed about the celebrities he had encountered, he almost always added a caveat that, ultimately, he didn't really care what they thought of him. "Why should I care what they think?" he said. "I'm in the entertainment business, and my photographs have entertained millions of people all over the world. Of course, each picture only entertains people for a few seconds. Even so, if you add all those seconds up, it's not *Gone with the Wind* or *Citizen Kane,* but it brings people joy."

Several months after my visit with Russell Turiak, I got a chance to talk on the phone with one of my longtime heroes, "the Edge," who is the lead guitarist for the band U2. His ambivalence about celebrity struck me immediately. "After our *Joshua Tree* album, we were as famous as you could be in music," he said, "and frankly, it was kind of overpowering for a while, but it really wasn't that interesting. If anything, it was something we tried to downplay. I don't think we ever *really* wanted celebrity, in and of itself, because we came out of the whole punk-rock thing, which was all about tearing that system down."

More than anything else, he said, fame was a kind of psychological torment for the band, especially in the beginning.

"Early on, we were kind of overwhelmed by it," he explained. "At the big U2 concerts we were really just hanging on to make it through. There was an element of desperation in which we were just trying to focus on our music. And if we got seduced by fame, I think our version of that was being too self-conscious, taking ourselves a little too seriously, and wondering, *Did we measure up? Were we a good enough band? Were we really able to do this?*" According to the Edge, fame's effect on the band was the opposite of a high—it induced a kind of low in which they constantly questioned themselves. Apparently, it had taken them years to outgrow this.

"I think now we are a little older, and we don't beat ourselves up quite so much," he said. "We feel extremely fortunate to have such great fans and to have written some great songs. Now, without being complacent, we're really enjoying what we're doing in a way that we probably wouldn't have earlier on, when there was an element of struggle, and nothing was ever good enough. We were always trying to reach beyond our abilities. We still do that now, but we also accept that we have certain limitations. It just gets to a point where you go, 'This is me. I am not everything I would like to be as an artist, but that doesn't mean I don't have anything worth saying.' "

We chatted about celebrity and the emptiness of fame for almost an hour. The irony of this whole episode was that as soon as our conversation was over, I felt compelled to call a number of my friends and tell them I had just talked with the Edge. I was especially excited because he had offered me two tickets and backstage passes for U2's concert in Boston the following evening. For the next thirty-six hours I actually walked around under the blissful delusion that he and I were on the verge of becoming pals. On some level I realized that I was falling into the very trap I was meant to be objectively observing, but it made no difference. In my heart I admit that I felt thrilled, privileged, and special.

The following evening, before the concert started, I made my way backstage. It was a mob scene. The small concrete room was crawling with people—doctors, business executives, school-teachers, fashion models, and more than a few squealing children, all of whom had a connection to someone in the band. Needless to say, I never got even close to the Edge. I felt completely deflated. I also worried about what I would say to the friends I'd told about my budding rapport with him. Eventually I shook off my malaise, and enjoyed one of the best concerts I've ever attended. Still, somewhere deep down, well beyond the reach of rational thought, lurked a hunger that left me feeling supremely uncomfortable.

Why was I so desperate to talk to the Edge that night? For that matter, why did people in general pine to bond with and befriend celebrities? The answer may be found in something called Belongingness Theory. Some research psychologists have come to believe that the need to belong is every bit as urgent as the need for food and shelter. Supporters of this theory contend that the desire to belong is actually humankind's driving psychological force. As they see it, Freudian theories about sexuality are compelling, but not nearly as important as the primal yearning for social acceptance.

Belongingness Theory is rooted in evolution. It holds that humans who formed groups in ancient times increased their chances of survival and reproduction. When it came to hunting large animals or defending the campfire against marauders, groups fared better. Anthropologists point out that groups were resilient in a way that individuals weren't, because their members could spread out and offer a number of services, such as hunting, firewood gathering, and even healing. Groups are especially important for children. Those who stayed close to the group probably received more food, care, and protection. Perhaps most important, at least in terms of evolution, adults in groups were more likely to find mates, reproduce, and form long-term parental relationships, increasing the chances that their children would reach maturity and reproduce themselves.

Belongingness Theory posits that over time, evolution has

created a sort of internal mechanism that makes us crave social acceptance. This mechanism prompts us to feel stressed when we are isolated and pleased when we interact with others. Some psychologists, including Jaak Panksepp, of the Medical College of Ohio at Toledo, claim that the formation of social relationships actually stimulates the production of opioids—chemicals in the brain that make us feel pleasure. Panksepp goes so far as to say that "social affect and social bonding are in some fundamental neurochemical sense opioid addictions." In other words, what started as a basic survival mechanism has evolved into an addiction to natural chemicals that our bodies release whenever we socialize.

This has direct implications for how we react to famous actors and even to the fictional characters they portray on television and in the movies. I've always been a fan of the TV show *Cheers*. In fact, not far from where I live in Boston, there is a sign for the bar Cheers, and I'm frequently tempted to stop in and have a beer at the place where Norm, Cliff, Carla, and Sam hung out—only it's not the place where they hung out, because *that place* never really even existed except on some Hollywood back lot.

Evidently, I've formed what research psychologists call a "para-social" relationship with the characters on the show. The notion of such a relationship was first discussed by two psychologists, Donald Horton and R. Richard Wohl, in a 1956 article for the journal *Psychiatry*. They argued that television gives viewers "the illusion of a face-to-face relationship with the performer." Over the course of many episodes, viewers come to feel that they know a given performer or a fictional persona. Horton and Wohl write:

> The persona offers, above all, a continuing relationship. His appearance is a regular and dependable event, to be counted on, planned for, and integrated into the routines of daily life. His devotees "live with him" and share the small episodes of his public life—and to some extent even of his private life away from the show. Indeed, their continued association with him

acquires a history . . . In time, the devotee—the "fan"—comes to believe that he "knows" the persona more intimately and profoundly than others do.

There are numerous examples of this phenomenon. Soap-opera viewers send flowers and condolence cards to TV studios when a favorite character is injured or killed in a tragic episode. Hordes of "Trekkies" obsess over Captain Kirk, Mr. Spock, and the other fictional personae on *Star Trek.* Perhaps the most extreme example involves Robert Young, the actor who starred in the series *Marcus Welby, MD.* In the early 1970s, during his first five years on the show, he received some 250,000 letters from viewers, most of them asking for medical advice.

One important thing that has changed since the 1950s, when Horton and Wohl introduced their theory, is that we (the public) can now know as much about the personal lives of our favorite stars as we do about the fictional lives they portray on TV and in the movies. In the early 2000s, for example, fans could follow the romantic entanglements of Rachel Green on the TV show *Friends,* and they could also then watch *Access Hollywood,* or pick up a copy of *Us Weekly,* to catch up on the love life of Jennifer Aniston, who played Rachel. According to Robert Thompson, of Syracuse University, the upshot of this is it is now easier than ever to form para-social relationships—not just with fictional personae but with actual celebrities as well. It all comes down to access, Thompson says, and the venues that offer glimpses into the lives of celebrities—magazines, books, Web sites, online chat rooms, radio and TV talk shows—seem endless.

"Just look at the rise in TV talk shows," Thompson says. "In the sixties you had just a few TV talk-show hosts, like Johnny Carson and Dick Cavett, who interviewed celebrities, whereas nowadays—especially with cable and satellite channels—you've got dozens of these hosts interviewing every last celebrity. You've got Oprah Winfrey, David Letterman, Jay Leno, Carson Daly, Conan O'Brien, Ellen DeGeneres, Jon Stewart, Martha

Stewart, Jenny Jones, Jimmy Kimmel, Montel Williams, Maury Povich, Jerry Springer, Ricki Lake, Rosie O'Donnell, Sally Jessy Raphael, Tony Danza, Tyra Banks—and the list goes on." All these hosts offer us a chance to meet celebrities "being themselves," he says.

Another major change since the 1950s is that Americans now appear to be lonelier than ever. In his book *The Loss of Happiness in Market Democracies,* the Yale political scientist Robert Lane notes that the number of people who described themselves as lonely more than quadrupled in the past few decades. We have increasingly become a nation of loners—traveling salesmen, Web designers, phone-bank operators, and on-line day traders who live and work in isolation. According to the U.S. Census Bureau, we also marry later in life. In 1956 the median age for marriage was 22.5 for men and 20.1 for women; by 2004 it was 27.4 for men and 25.8 for women. This helps to explain something else the Census Bureau has noted: Americans are increasingly living alone. The share of American households including seven or more people dropped from 35.9 percent in 1790, 5.8 percent in 1950, and 1.2 percent in 2004. Meanwhile, the number of households consisting of just one person rose from 3.7 percent in 1790 to 9.3 percent in 1950 and 26.4 percent in 2004. Nowadays, one out of four American households consists of a single person. In recent years this trend has been especially discernible among young people. Since 1970 the number of youths (ages fifteen to twenty-five) living alone has almost tripled, and the number of young adults (ages twenty-five to thirty-four) living alone has more than quadrupled.

The combination of loneliness and our innate desire to belong may be fueling our interest in celebrities and our tendency to form para-social relationships with them. Only a few research psychologists have seriously explored this possibility, among them Lynn McCutcheon and Dianne Ashe. McCutcheon and Ashe compared results from 150 subjects who had taken three personality tests—one measuring shyness, one measuring loneliness, and one measuring celebrity obsession, on something called the Celebrity Attitudes Scale, or CAS. The CAS asks subjects to rate the veracity of statements such as "I am obsessed by details of my favorite celebrity's life" and "If I were lucky enough to meet my favorite celebrity, and he/she asked me to do something illegal as a favor, I would probably do it." McCutcheon and Ashe found a correlation among scores on loneliness, shyness, and the CAS. Their results led McCutcheon to observe in a subsequent paper, "Perhaps one of the ways [we] cope with shyness and loneliness is to cultivate a 'safe,' non-threatening relationship with a celebrity."

Another investigation, led by Jacki Fitzpatrick, of Texas Tech University, looked at the correlation between para-social relationships and actual romantic relationships. Fitzpatrick asked forty-five college students to complete a questionnaire containing several psychological measures, including one that gauged para-social relationships (the Para-social Interaction Scale) and another that gauged romantic relationships (the Multiple Determinants of Relationship Commitment Inventory). She and her colleague, Andrea McCourt, discovered that subjects who were less invested in their romantic relationships were more involved in para-social relationships. They concluded, "It makes sense that individuals may use para-social relationships as one way to fulfill desires or address needs (e.g., for attention, companionship) that are unmet in their romances."

The Rochester survey, too, provides evidence that lonely teenagers are especially susceptible to forming para-social relationships with celebrities. Boys who described themselves as lonely were almost twice as likely as others to endorse the statement "My favorite celebrity just helps me feel good and forget about all of my troubles." Girls who described themselves as lonely were almost three times as likely as others to endorse that statement.

Another survey question asked teens whom they would most like to meet for dinner: Jesus Christ, Albert Einstein, Shaquille O'Neal, Jennifer Lopez, 50 Cent, Paris Hilton, or President Bush. Among boys who said they were not lonely, the clear winner was Jesus Christ; but among those who described themselves as lonely, Jesus finished last and 50 Cent was the clear winner. Similarly, girls who felt appreciated by their parents, friends, and teachers tended to choose dinner with Jesus, whereas those who felt underappreciated were likely to choose Paris Hilton. One possible interpretation of these results is that lonely and underappreciated teens particularly want to befriend the ultimate popular guy or girl.

In Russell Turiak's generation, that guy was Steve McQueen; nowadays he appears to be 50 Cent. Regardless of who exactly this figure is at a given time, it's clear that many of us—lonely people in particular—yearn to belong to the popular crowd. And perhaps what really separates most of us from someone like Russell Turiak is that he actually tries to infiltrate that crowd, while the rest of us simply enjoy this experience, once removed, through his pictures.

Around the time I met Russell Turiak, I also got to know a Hollywood publicist named Michael Levine. I'd first seen Levine on television as Michael Jackson's publicist during Jackson's first child-molestation scandal, in the early 1990s. He'd been in the business more than twenty years, representing quite a few stars, and had written a number of books on public relations, including *Charming Your Way to the Top: Hollywood's Premier PR Executive Shows You How to Get Ahead,* and *Raise Your Social I.Q: How to Do the Right Thing in Any Situation.*

Levine and I met for tea one afternoon at the Century Plaza Hotel in Los Angeles. We found each other in the hotel's soaring, sun-drenched lobby, where a pianist in a tuxedo played soft jazz while a svelte waitress whose nametag read "Queenie" served drinks to tourists laden with Gucci and Versace shopping bags. Levine was a tall, handsome man in his midfifties with watery blue eyes, an aquiline nose, and a shock of gray hair slicked back with gel.

When we shook hands, he greeted me loudly, as if he were greeting everyone in our section of the lobby. I quickly discovered that Levine had two modes of speaking. The first was his broadcast mode, in which he spoke with the volume and authority of a courtroom lawyer. The second was his intimate mode, in which he drew close, made unwavering eye contact, and spoke in a hushed manner as if letting me in on a secret that was far too sensitive for public consumption. His intimate voice was rare, and when he used it, I had the impression I might be speaking with Michael Levine the person.

"Are you familiar with my Tiffany's theory?" he asked as we sat down.

I told him I wasn't.

Levine cleared his throat and explained. "If I visit you today and give you a present, and I give it to you in a Tiffany's box, in your mind the gift that I gave you has a higher perceived value than if I gave it to you in *no* box or a box of lesser prestige. The reason that's true is not because you are a psychological jackass"—he smiled briefly, presumably to convey that no offense was intended—"but because you and I and your wife and this waitress live in a culture in which we gift-wrap everything. We gift-wrap our politicians, our corporate heads, our TV and movie stars, and even our toilet paper."

"So you see yourself as gift-wrapping celebrities?"

"Yes," he replied. "That is the analogy."

When I asked him to clarify one aspect of his theory, he responded by asking which of the ninety-nine words I wanted him to repeat. I said I'd like to hear the entire theory again. Levine nodded, gathered himself for a minute, and then repeated his words verbatim, with the same seemingly nonchalant facial expressions and hand gestures he'd used before. Clearly, this was a man who had perfected the art of speaking in sound bites; I began to worry that he wasn't going to tell me anything he hadn't already composed, edited, and delivered dozens of times before.

Nonetheless, I pressed on, and asked Levine how he had become, as his books claimed, "Hollywood's premier PR executive."

"The arc of anyone's career . . . ," he began, and then paused to reconsider his approach. "Scratch that," he said. "Yours is a multidimensional question. Is it luck? Is it timing? Is it skill? I'm not sure, but I have represented some of the most successful people in the world." He paused again and then rattled off the following names in rapid-fire succession: "Michael Jackson, Charlton Heston, Nancy Kerrigan, Demi Moore, Michael J. Fox, Sandra Bullock, David Bowie, Prince, Kareem Abdul-Jabbar, Jon Stewart, Dave Chappelle, Cameron Diaz, Bill O'Reilly, Ozzy Osbourne, Bob Evans, and Barbra Streisand. I learned something very important when I was working for Barbra Streisand on New Year's Eve. It was an event at the MGM in Las Vegas, and she hadn't performed in many years—two decades, actually—and right at midnight, or perhaps twelve-thirty, she asked me whether I could find her some plum sauce. Plum sauce—like you get in a Chinese restaurant. And I figured something out real quick. When Barbra Streisand asks you for plum sauce on New Year's Eve in Las Vegas, 'No' is a really bad answer. And 'I don't know' is a really bad answer. 'Yes,' however, is a really good answer. You've got to figure that out! And the higher you get, the harder it gets. The demands get more intensified."

I asked him how he, as a professional at the top of his field, coped with such demands.

"This is a question that goes through your head at the beginning of your career," he admitted in a quiet voice. "But I want you to understand: Getting someone plum sauce in Las Vegas at midnight on New Year's Eve is challenging, but it's not murder. It's not so ludicrous. And professionals who work at the top of their field in the fame game realize that this is simply part of the game."

In the end, Levine said, any misgivings he had about occasionally being asked to fetch plum sauce were far outweighed by the status he gained in performing such duties. "Look," he said, "I've seen strangers look at Mike Tyson and say, 'What a scumbag, what a vermin, what a douche bag.' Then, as he gets closer, they start getting excited. And then, three minutes later, they want their picture taken with him. Fame is a validator. The conflict is that I want it. You want it. We all want it—or want to be close to it. But what is the price? It's the Faustian bargain. You see what I mean? Celebrities offer you the drug of validation, but you can't talk straight to the pusher, or you won't get your drug. That's the deal."

Hollywood, like Washington, D.C., is known for being an insular company town where everybody competes for recognition, status, and, above all, proximity. In Washington it is commonly said that your status can be measured by how many degrees of separation exist between you and the president; in Hollywood the same is often said of Jack Nicholson or Steven Spielberg.

One could argue that this fight for proximity, in which we strive to ingratiate ourselves with famous and prestigious people, goes well beyond those power vortexes and plays itself out in many corners of America. Perhaps the best example of this can be found in studies on the social dynamics of cheerleaders. According to the sociologists Pamela Bettis and Natalie Adams, 3.3 million people participate in cheerleading each year. They observe, "Numerous scholars have documented that cheerleading is often perceived as the highest-status activity for girls in middle school, and girls who cheer often occupy positions of power, prestige, and privilege in their schools."

In a landmark study Donna Eder examined the social dynamics of cheerleaders at an unspecified middle school in the Midwest. Eder and several research assistants spent more than a year interviewing students during lunch, between classes, and at special after-school events such as dances and picnics. In the process Eder identified an elite group—composed primarily of cheerleaders—that most of the other girls wanted to join. The members of this elite group were typically referred to as the "popular girls" by the rest of the students. According to Eder, these girls commanded the school's attention. Eder observed that girls throughout the school discussed the activities of the popular girls, but the popular girls paid almost no attention to anyone but themselves. She also noted that non-cheerleaders often went to great lengths to ingratiate themselves with the cheerleaders:

> Many of the girls wanted to sit with the cheerleaders at lunch and made special attempts to be friendly toward them. For example, when it looked as though cheerleading might be eliminated from the school budget, Sylvia made a point of telling Carrie, one of the new cheerleaders, that she had written a letter to President Reagan telling him how important cheerleading was for school spirit and how hard some of her friends had worked to become cheerleaders. Also, if one of the new cheerleaders was upset about something, there were usually many girls around to comfort her.

Eder concluded that there were "two main avenues for mobility into the elite group—becoming a cheerleader or becoming a friend of a cheerleader." But few cheerleading positions were ever available, so all the other girls engaged in a desperate race to befriend the school's pompom-toting elite. The upshot of all this, observed Eder, is that teenage girls often become more self-conscious and preoccupied with being liked.

The social lives of cheerleaders and celebrities are strikingly similar. Both groups consist of and are defined by two types of people: the "stars," who appear talented, glamorous, and popular; and the "acolytes," who strive to endear themselves to the stars. The question is: What exactly motivates the acolytes? To a certain extent, Belongingness Theory explains why so many of us yearn to belong to groups in general, but not why we prefer these highly prestigious groups above all others, or why we toil to ingratiate ourselves with the leaders of these groups.

Francisco Gil-White, an evolutionary anthropologist at the University of Pennsylvania, offers one explanation. In 2001 he and a colleague, Joseph Henrich, of Emory University, proposed the idea of Prestige Theory. The core of the theory is based on the notion that humans—unlike chimps, orangutans, and other primates—have the unique ability to learn and perfect highly nuanced skills. Perhaps the best example of this involves an experiment conducted by two Emory primatologists, Josep Call and Michael Tomasello, who tested and compared the learning abilities of adult orangutans and four-year-old humans. According to Call and Tomasello, orangutans have a reputation among primatologists for being skillful problem solvers. To test just how clever they were, the researchers built a small contraption that dispensed M&M chocolate candies. It had a long steel handle that could be pushed, pulled, or rotated. During the experiment a researcher would manipulate the handle in a combination of ways, and if the orangutan successfully mimicked this motion, it received an M&M. Call and Tomasello discovered that the adult orangutans were not nearly as successful as the four-year-old humans at doing this. They concluded that orangutans "did not use imitative learning to help them solve the problem presented," whereas children "did use their observations of the demonstrations to help them solve the task."

Gil-White and Henrich relied on experiments like this one to argue that only humans have the ability to observe and then mimic complex behaviors. They claim that this uniquely human ability eventually created "prestige hierarchies" in which those with the most valuable skills sat at the top. So when a truly talented hunter emerged in prehistoric times, he was revered both because he brought home food and because his skill could be learned. Disciples soon gravitated toward this hunter. They "paid" for access by doing favors for him, excusing him from certain obligations, and siding with him politically. Posses of studious disciples eventually formed. According to Gil-White and Henrich, these posses served as beacons, allowing hungry tribe members to identify a mentor, learn a skill, and begin feeding themselves as quickly as possible.

The premise of Prestige Theory is that it has been evolutionarily advantageous for human beings to identify prestigious people and befriend them in order to gain skills. In ancient times the disciple of a successful hunter stood a better chance of surviving, having children, and then feeding them. By this rationale, over the millennia astute disciples have flourished. But perhaps even more interesting is the notion that human beings have developed a conditioned response to entourages. In theory, at least, we are genetically predisposed to identifying posses of admirers and gravitating toward the leaders (or people with the skills) because historically this is how our ancestors survived and reproduced. So when Michael Levine fetches plum sauce for Barbra Streisand, or Sylvia tries to ingratiate herself with a "skilled" cheerleader, the invisible hand of evolution is simply pushing them along.

These instincts still help us in modern-day scenarios. In many work settings, for example, it pays to identify and endear oneself to the man or woman at the center of a posse of admirers. This allows one to learn valuable skills—today's equivalent of hunting school. But according to Gil-White, whom I interviewed, this goes all wrong when it comes to celebrities. When we see them on TV, we sense that they are at the center of a truly enormous entourage, so our conditioned "posse response" is activated, and we gravitate toward them. A few savvy operators, like Michael Levine, can actually find their way into the posse and become disciples or insiders. The overwhelming majority of us, however, can't. And we are the real losers in this scenario because we subconsciously attempt to ingratiate ourselves with our idols—buying Paris Hilton's jewelry and Nicole Kidman's perfume—without really gaining anything. In essence we are still chasing the great hunters; but, of course, most of these hunters have no interest in teaching us, and worse yet, many of them have little of real value to teach.

Whatever motivated Michael Levine to run errands for his famous clients, he at least had the satisfaction of knowing that he had been invited to the party. Russell Turiak did not. Turiak made this point to me toward the end of my visit with him in Yonkers. He did it in a roundabout manner, by inviting me to see one final photograph that he especially treasured—a large framed picture of Hulk Hogan and Shaquille O'Neal. This was somehow different from all the other photos of his that I'd seen. In a minute I realized why: it was posed. When I mentioned this, Turiak smiled and said that he'd actually been *asked* to take it. The invitation came from a promoter who had arranged a fight between Hogan and Rick Flair, for which O'Neal would be the referee. The promoter wanted a shot of Shaq and Hulk standing together. Turiak wouldn't be paid for his work, but when the shoot was over, he would be free to sell his extras.

We stood silently admiring the photo. Finally Turiak asked if I was familiar with James Lipton and the show *Inside the Actors Studio*. I nodded. I had watched Lipton interview a number of famous actors. "Okay, good," Turiak said. "Now, you know the part where he asks the questions like 'What's your favorite curse word?' 'What sound do you love to hear?' 'What sound do you hate to hear?' And then the last question is 'If there is a heaven, when you get there, what would you like to hear them say?' Well sometimes I imagine myself answering this question, and my reply is always 'Your name is on the list.'"

For a moment Turiak simply stared at me and smiled, but it was an odd, mirthless smile that seemed stretched a bit too tightly, and it gave me an uneasy feeling.

"But you know what?" he said. "If my name isn't on the list, I'll just find a way to go around the back and sneak in—because *that* is what I do."

When Reflected Glory Isn't Enough: Confessions of an Upwardly Mobile Celebrity "Slave"

O NE EVENING MICHAEL LEVINE invited me to dinner to continue our conversation about celebrities and those who served them. We met at a small Italian restaurant alongside a toupee shop and a chiropractor's office, on the sort of strip-mall-laden L.A. boulevard that never makes it into the movies. Over dinner Levine talked at length about why fame held such allure for him, and eventually he related much of this to his childhood.

"You have to bear in mind that when I was growing up, I never knew anyone who owned a tuxedo," he told me. His family had never had a color TV, and he had not attended college. In general, he had almost nothing good to say about his childhood. He described his mother as an alcoholic and his father as "a good but very passive, weak man whose whole orientation was to avoid conflict." That said, he blamed his parents for nothing; rather, he credited them for instilling in him a "burning, maniacal rage" to succeed.

"Usually there is some searing experience in our childhood, sometimes humorously described as the guy who doesn't get the girls in high school, that prompts us to work hard and compensate," he said. "Perhaps in my case this searing experience derived from the fact that I—like Bill Clinton and other children of alcoholics—grew up feeling like an inherent, internal piece of shit. So I tried to push ahead. And in American life today maybe a currency worth more than money is fame." One of the best things about fame, he concluded, is its fluidity; to some extent its prestige simply flows from one person to another. The best example of this, he insisted, was his Mike Tyson anecdote. Tyson was reviled by a great many people, but ultimately it didn't matter, because he was still a bona fide celebrity, and anyone who got near him could, as Levine put it, "bask in his reflected glory."

Over the past several decades research psychologists have explored the concept of reflected glory. One of the first to do so was Robert Cialdini, now a professor of psychology at Arizona State University. In the mid-1970s Cialdini was teaching at Ohio State University when he noticed one day that virtually everyone on campus was wearing an OSU Windbreaker or sweatshirt. He told me, "I had no idea what was going on until I learned that the school's football team had just been ranked number one in the country. It seemed to me that everyone was literally dressing themselves in the success of the team." This observation eventually prompted Cialdini to conduct a study in which a team of investigators monitored how students dressed at seven universities with well-regarded football teams. Every Monday, Cialdini's investigators attended Introduction to Psychology classes and counted the students wearing clothes emblazoned with the school's name or logo. Without fail, when a school's football team had won a game the previous Saturday, more students wore school apparel. Cialdini concluded that when a team lost, students tended to distance themselves from that failure, but when it won, they reveled in the victory as if it were their own. He called this "basking in reflected glory," or "BIRGing."

Cialdini soon began investigating what types of people were most likely to BIRG. He suspected that those with low self-esteem—especially if their self-esteem had recently been diminished—would be the likeliest. He tested his theory in an experiment in which he and his researchers randomly telephoned students at Arizona State and asked them to participate in a trivia quiz about their school. The researchers told half the students that they had done very well on the quiz, and the other half that they had done very poorly. The same students were then asked to describe how ASU's football team had fared on a particular Saturday. The results showed that students tended to use the pronoun "we" in describing a victory and "they" in describing a defeat—and this tendency was strongest among students who had just "failed" the trivia quiz. Cialdini concluded that students with low or diminished self-esteem were looking for a way to salvage their reputations or sense of self, and often did so by basking in the reflected glory of their team when it won.

Eventually Cialdini came to believe that his findings on the relationship between BIRGing and self-esteem might apply to a number of situations outside the realm of sports. To test this he conducted an experiment in which he administered a fake personality test that allegedly measured social skills. He told half his subjects that they had scored well on this test, and the other half that they had scored poorly. Then he had all the students read one of two articles. The first was about an intelligent student named Douglas Schofield who had a promising future; the second was about an unsuccessful student named Douglas Schofield who was on the verge of dropping out of school. Both articles contained a lot of details about Schofield, including his date of birth. Unbeknownst to the subjects in this study, Cialdini had customized every single article so that Schofield always had the same birthday as the reader. Afterward Cialdini and his assistants asked all the subjects what they made of this coincidence. Subjects who'd been told that they had scored poorly on their personality tests typically went out of their way either to associate themselves with the "intelligent" Schofield or to distance themselves from the "unintelligent" Schofield. Cialdini concluded that those whose self-esteem had been diminished were more likely to embrace connections to successful people and distance themselves from unsuccessful people.

Of course, Cialdini's findings aren't all that surprising. It seems commonsensical that people who feel bad about themselves—and even many who don't—would want to enhance their self-esteem by associating with famous or successful people. What is surprising is that these people would be so eager to BIRG that they would latch on to such a trivial and tenuous connection as a shared birthday. In light of this, it makes perfect sense that fans would stand in the pouring rain for hours to catch a glimpse of a movie star, or that a Hollywood professional would do any number of menial tasks just to maintain a connection with a celebrity. After all, as Cialdini points out, even the slightest connection can be a useful vehicle for BIRGing.

Although dozens of studies have been done on how BIRGing works in the sports world, almost none have been done on how it might apply to the world of Hollywood celebrities. The closest thing may be another study Cialdini conducted involving birthdays. There was no self-esteem component to this study, but its results were intriguing. Cialdini asked his subjects to read a short biography of Grigori Rasputin, the notorious monk who served as an adviser in the court of Czar Nicolas II, and to give their opinion of him. The biography depicted Rasputin as a mendacious and manipulative villain. In half the cases Cialdini had adjusted Rasputin's birthday so that it matched that of the reader. Those subjects who shared a birthday with Rasputin were overwhelmingly more likely to rate him positively—as a strong and effective leader with many redeeming qualities. Cialdini calls this "boosting." Basically, when we boost, we try to make ourselves feel better by bolstering the reputation of a highly visible person, team, or institution to which we are already connected.

"What it all comes down to is that most of us want to make a positive connection to great people," Cialdini told me. "And you can do this by actively creating a connection to someone who is great, or, if you already have that connection, you can boost that person's image so it becomes more positive—even if that person is someone as reviled as Grigori Rasputin." What's more, having made a connection to a "great" person, we will go out of our way to flatter and aggrandize that person—not necessarily because we like being obsequious but because subconsciously this boosts our *own* self-esteem. According to Cialdini, the process is intensified in a city like L.A., where connections to the famous are so highly valued. "I used to live in L.A.," he said, "and I remember you couldn't go into a restaurant or a store without seeing framed pictures of the celebrities who frequented that place. The ethos of BIRGing was so deeply ingrained in the psyche of the city that even my local dry cleaner was getting caught up in it."

As my dinner with Michael Levine neared its end, a question lingered in my mind: How did a well-respected professional like him, who associated with many famous people and received a great deal of reflected glory, check his own desire to become famous? When I asked, Levine nodded excitedly. "It's a constant concern," he said. "I just met these two producers at the Beverly Wilshire Hotel, and they proposed that we do a reality-TV show called *Hollywood Boot Camp*. The idea is this: Interns from around the world come to Hollywood, where celebrities give them team assignments and I am the drill sergeant. I am the Lou Gossett Jr. character from *An Officer and a Gentleman*." Levine went on to weigh the pros and cons of participating in *Hollywood Boot Camp*, but his musings all seemed to lead to a single question: "What will this do for my obituary?"

"After all," he said, "Charlton Heston fucked up his obituary. I worked for him for eighteen years, and in the end he became a cult member for the National Rifle Association. When Heston got into the NRA, I could see that those people were manipulating him. Before that, his obituary would have read that he was a legendary film star—now he is a gun-rights nut. Likewise, I would become a cartoon character. People don't consider what impact the things they do have on their tombstone or obituary. They are always focused on the immediate." According to Levine, he was constantly being called upon by the media to comment on various celebrity-related issues. "If I wanted to, I could be on national TV twice a week for the rest of my life," he said.

A few days later I happened to be with him when he received

some breaking news on the Martha Stewart trial. "Whenever there is a major incident involving a celebrity, I get calls from CNN, MSNBC, CNBC, or Fox News," he told me, as we hopped into a limo and whizzed across town toward a television studio so he could partake in yet another such interview. "After all, the networks have twenty-four hours of news to fill." Levine had written a book on branding, *A Branded World,* and a number of TV news producers wanted him to comment on the Martha Stewart trial. "Basically, if you say something with modesty and lucidity, it will help you," he told me. "But there are people who overuse their media access. The problem is that it's hard to know whether you are giving a speech because you want to affect 'the dialogue' or because you want to hear the roar of the crowd. It's all very seductive. Someone from Fox News will call and say, 'There are all these crazies on TV talking about Michael Jackson, but you are a cut above. Your mind is needed here. You can add to the dialogue.' And of course that's a rush—but you have to check it."

At the studio a makeup artist greeted Levine warmly and immediately began fussing with his hair and smearing foundation across his cheeks and brow. "What's the topic today?" he asked, stroking Levine's face with a small brush.

"Martha Stewart on MSNBC."

"Oh," said the makeup artist without much enthusiasm. He turned to me and said, "Michael and I have been through it all: Martha Stewart, Michael Jackson, Kobe Bryant, Princess Di—the list goes on."

During the interview, as Levine offered a few sound bites about the damage that had been done to Martha Stewart's brand, I was reminded of Robert Thompson, of Syracuse University. This was precisely the sort of interview Thompson often did, though he, too, was leery of getting too comfortable in the spotlight. "All this being on television is highly suspect to an academic," Thompson told me during one of our discussions. "We get to justify it because we are trying to explore fame and the media and understand how it works. The problem is that we're getting a certain degree of fame ourselves, and we are really just feeding from this frenzy like everyone else." The key was to pull back occasionally, Thompson had concluded, so he sometimes forced himself to turn down interviews. "Otherwise you can get overexposed, and you'll be taken less seriously if you look like you are constantly available to talk about anything."

Ultimately, it was a similar set of concerns that prompted Levine to turn down the offer from the producers of *Hollywood Boot Camp.* By making these decisions, both men had exercised restraint, which no doubt boded well for their obituaries. But what about those insiders who didn't check themselves, and instead tried to soak up every last errant ray of the spotlight?

Marcel Winter has made a life for himself by dressing other people, mainly celebrities—Halle Berry, Jim Carrey, John Travolta, and Nicole Kidman among them. Over the years, Winter has also developed a successful second career as an analyst of celebrity fashion for several television networks, identifying the best- and worst-dressed attendees at events like the Oscars and the Golden Globes. Indeed, Winter has used his status as a celebrity stylist to jump-start a booming cottage industry in which he has written magazine articles, authored a book, designed a line of jewelry for QVC, and been a spokesman for products including razor blades, luxury cars, fast food, and toothpaste.

After submitting an interview request to one of his assistants, I received an e-mail containing instructions worthy of an Ian Fleming novel: I was to go to Central Park in Manhattan at 11:30 and sit on a bench at the East 72nd Street entrance. There I would be met by a man with a cane.

On the appointed day I waited for Winter at the specified bench in Central Park. Almost half an hour passed. Finally I saw a blind man approaching with a rickety collapsible cane. As he drew closer, the man said, "Are you the writer?"

"Yes," I replied.

"I can kind of see you. I'm Marcel Winter."

He sat down on the bench next to me. He was wearing camouflage Reebok sneakers, brown cargo pants, and a well-worn T-shirt that read "Africa Is Our Home." He was extremely thin, with wispy brown hair and long arms lined with sinewy muscles and bulging green veins.

"I'm not completely blind," Winter said, in what sounded like a Maine accent. "Many people who are blind can see in a limited way. For example, I can see that cars are passing and that a woman over there who just walked past is wearing something bright, like purple."

"Have you been blind your entire life?" I asked.

"No, man, I'm a stylist! I need my eyes—I'm just studying for a part in a movie!" Suddenly his Maine accent disappeared, and in its place came a thick New York accent. "The character in the movie is blind, so I wear these contact lenses that purposely fuck up my vision. I play the role of a blind man from Maine named Daniel Moody who talks like this . . ." Winter paused, and then he was back in character. "I'm real quiet, and I get beaten up, and I wear clothing that feels good, but I am blind, so the clothes don't match. You may notice that I also rock a lot." He bobbed his head back and forth in a vaguely Ray Charles manner. Winter said this movie was the "opportunity of a lifetime," because it gave him his first chance to play a leading role in an actual film. (I later learned that it was a low-budget independent film about a blind man who attempts to leave his home after decades of living in isolation.) Winter had previously appeared in some TV specials about fashion, in which he had played himself, but as far as he was concerned, this was his first foray into acting.

"When I'm acting, it's almost like I'm channeling Daniel," he told me. He found the role refreshing, because Daniel was a person who just said what he thought in a blunt, childlike manner. "When you're wearing the stylist's hat, you can't be so outspoken," Winter said. "As a stylist, you have to learn to be very diplomatic and say the right things, especially with celebrities."

He began digging into his pockets for a pack of cigarettes and a lighter, which he eventually found. Awkwardly he pulled out a cigarette and put it in his mouth, and made several fumbling attempts to light it. "This is difficult," he grumbled. "I guess this is why blind people don't smoke—they'd burn their noses off."

When he had finally lit the cigarette, Winter took a long drag and leaned back against the bench. I asked him to tell me about his work as a stylist.

"Well," he said, "I'll spend days dressing people for events I dress myself for in five minutes." The bulk of his job, it seemed, was to play the role of court jester. It usually took him only about thirty minutes to dress a celebrity for an event, but he would often end up staying as long as nine hours in order to entertain them, fuss over them, and listen to them complain. "It's very disconcerting," he said, "because you invest so much of your time, and you really become their slave. I don't mean it in a bad sense, by any means—you just have to be there for them, and it's just interesting that they don't take the time to do the same for you." According to Winter, in all his years of work, only once had a client had the decency to notify him that she would be leaving him for another stylist. "It's sad, because you think you're friends with them," he told me, "but now I know that it's just work and it's not personal."

Rather abruptly, Winter jerked his head around and asked, "What's that over there?"

I turned and saw that a large wedding party had just finished posing for pictures in the park. "It's a wedding," I said. "The bride and groom are actually walking toward us."

"I love going to weddings," Winter said. "It's the most exciting thing, to be a part of someone's personal history." Neither of us spoke as the wedding party drew near. When the bride and groom had passed, Winter rose to his feet and gestured for us to begin walking. I offered my arm for guidance. As we walked, he reminisced about the stars he had dressed, and how this had made him the most highly visible person in his field. "If you asked a hundred people on the street to name a stylist, eighty people would not be able to name anyone, and the other nineteen would name me. But I'm at the end of this phase of my career. I've given everyone in Hollywood their day, many days, and I've been blessed enough, but now I've got a chance to have that life—to become a celebrity."

When we reached the western edge of the park, Winter paused to get his bearings and then set off northward at a steady clip. As we walked, he explained that he was due at an acting lesson, which he invited me to attend. As we attempted to cross a busy intersection, he seemed to lose his patience and he stepped out into oncoming traffic, where he was almost flattened by a taxi. "It's amazing!" he said. "In this city the cabdrivers will just cut you off! And I'm like, 'Dude, I'm blind. If you hit me, I'm going to own your house.' But they're not thinking that. They're thinking, 'I'm going to get to that corner before the blind guy does. Fucking blind guy—run him over.' And I'm like, 'There's a five-foot cane with a red thing on it. You didn't notice that, dude?' People are just funny. I've been talking about Hollywood, but it's really the whole world. Everyone's a star in their own movie."

Winter and I made our way to a handsome brownstone on West 87th Street, where I met his acting coach, Heather Brills, a faculty member at the Yale School of Drama. Brills was a slender blonde dressed in a black leotard with a pink scarf wrapped around her waist. She led us through an opulent living room furnished with Persian carpets, Tiffany lamps, a marble fireplace, and a chandelier. Upstairs, in a small studio, Winter and Brills sat cross-legged on the floor. Winter shook his head once, almost a shiver, and began speaking in the voice of Daniel Moody.

"I haven't left my home in twenty-five years," he said, bobbing his head. "I am not very comfortable in public."

"Good," said Brills. "Let's read the scene where you go into the bar."

In this scene Daniel unknowingly walks into a diner and has a series of awkward encounters. After the reading Winter seemed quite pleased until he received his first suggestion. "Let's read it again," Brills said. "But this time let's have a little more spontaneity and honesty from Daniel."

Winter considered this, but then he shook his head. "The real problem is the script. The lines just don't feel like words that Daniel would actually say."

"How so?" Brills asked.

"They're too proper. Daniel's been locked in a house for twenty-five years, and he's from rural Maine, and I doubt he would say 'Do they have beer here?' He would say 'They have beer—don't they?'"

Tactfully Brills pointed out that if Winter ignored the script, he would throw off the other actors. He disagreed, insisting that when the other actors heard his complaints, they would rally to his cause. Brills nodded sympathetically and then suggested that he try the lines again. The two began reading the scene, but thirty seconds later Winter stopped midsentence and announced that he could not read the next line—"It smells good in here"—because it just wasn't believable. "Do you really think Daniel would talk like that?" he asked. "I think he would say 'Smells good here.'" Brills didn't react immediately. She stared at him blankly, perhaps hoping he would let it go, but he was actually just getting started. Over the next two hours Winter aired dozens of grievances, even about the music she had chosen to simulate background music in the diner.

At one point he complained that his lines always landed at page breaks, whereas the other characters' lines were always neatly contained on a single page. "Everything is against me! Am I wrong? Are my points about the script valid, or are they crazy?" Silence fell over the studio. Winter and I were now both looking at Brills, waiting for her to respond. I assumed that this was a scenario he knew quite well: he was using his leverage as the actor and the client to push the envelope and to see how much he could get away with.

Through it all Brills did her best to remain calm. Only once did she betray her true feelings—when Winter left the apartment in order to practice his lines while walking through a doorway, as called for by the script. The minute the door closed, Brills leaned against a wall, closed her eyes, rubbed her temples, and gave a deep sigh of frustration. A second later, the door clanked open and Heather was smiling brightly.

After my time with Marcel Winter, I thought about the fine line between reflected glory and actual fame, especially in the context of Hollywood. I eventually called Robert Thompson and told him about my encounters with Winter and Levine. Thompson quickly concluded that their stories—and his own—were essentially variations on the same theme. They weren't really about reflected glory, insisted Thompson, they were stories about men who were looking to maximize their *direct* glory by whatever means available. According to Thompson, if he and Levine appeared to be holding back at times, it was not because they didn't want attention but because they wanted only a certain kind of attention.

"I doubt that Michael Levine turned down that TV show, *Hollywood Boot Camp,* because he didn't want fame," Thompson said. "He turned it down because he was thinking several steps ahead, and he wanted a lasting, respectable sort of fame that would follow him into his obituary." Thompson admitted that his own reasons for holding back were carefully considered. His main concern was not, as he put it, for truth, beauty, or the betterment of humankind. "My main concern is that I don't want the overexposure to jeopardize my future chances of being on TV."

In a way, all of us who dance on the periphery of the celebrity world—whether they are publicists, paparazzi, media studies professors, or journalists like me—are flirting with the notion of being famous. Certainly, part of the allure is the rush that comes from being in front of the camera. But it goes beyond this. Rightly or wrongly, society rewards those who throw themselves into the fame machine and manage to siphon off a bit of fame for themselves. As Thompson eventually admitted, "I recognize that the reason I have the biggest office, an endowed chair, and a good salary has less to do with the books I have written and more to do with the fact that the university is as obsessed with attention as everyone else."

In my own case, I've been fascinated by the celebrity world since I was a kid. Ostensibly this curiosity led me to approach the subject as an objective observer. And yet, either consciously or subconsciously, perhaps I am just looking for the most expedient path into the limelight. On this point Thompson agreed emphatically.

"I remember, as a kid, watching the TV show *Nova* for the first time," he said. "I came to the conclusion that I wanted to be a scientist—not in order to do science, but so that I could be that guy on TV with his name on the screen. Even watching something as intellectual and unglamorous as *Nova,* I was still being lured into the deliciousness of fame. I had already decided how I was going to get a piece of it, even though I was a nerdy kid. As academics—or even journalists—we like to play that down, but I think what we do is really the ultimate scam: we get our own fame by trying to expose the neuroses and psyche of other people who want fame. But being a professor, this is the only possible route I have. At the age of forty-five, I know I can't sing, dance, or be a sports star."

PART III

THE WORLD OF
CELEBRITY WORSHIPERS

Monkeys, *Us Weekly,* and the
Power of Social Information

W HEN IT COMES to knowing exactly where celebrities live, there is no greater expert than Bill Gordon. His book, *The Ultimate Hollywood Tour Book,* has sold more than 40,000 copies and is considered to be the definitive celebrity atlas. Among other things, Gordon tells his readers when a given house was built, who its various owners have been, and how much it most recently sold for; sometimes his book reads like a reference sheet for real-estate agents. Gordon notes that Johnny Depp paid only $2.3 million for his twenty-nine-room mansion, because he bought it from a divorce lawyer who was convicted of tax fraud, whereas Nicholas Cage paid $6.5 million for a house with only four rooms more. He offers detailed directions for finding these places, complete with little asides ("Note: In what seems like a conspiracy to confuse tourists, Monovale Drive changes its name and becomes Carolwood Drive at this point"). Finally, Gordon issues a word of caution: "If you approach a celebrity at his or her home, he or she may construe the approach as a hostile act and act accordingly. Remember: not all celebrities are as volatile as Sean Penn or Sean Young. But why take a chance?"

I met Bill Gordon in front of the Beverly Hills Hotel on a perfectly sunny afternoon, and almost immediately our attention was distracted by a teenager just down the street who was selling star maps for $10 apiece. Gordon shook his head. "Most of the star maps that get sold on street corners haven't been updated," he said matter-of-factly. To prove his point, Gordon walked briskly toward the teenager and bought a map. At fifty-three, Gordon was the personification of good health; his black walking shorts and knee-high athletic socks gave him the look of a no-nonsense high school football coach marching down the field.

Opening the map, Gordon said, "Look at this! Here is Dan Aykroyd's house, even though he moved to New York City six years ago. These mapmakers simply take no pride in their work. They don't update their information, and they pawn their maps off as something they're not. It's just consumer fraud. When I see lazy maps like this, I do take offense." He quickly added that his book, currently in its nineteenth edition, was updated annually. He pores over newspaper clippings and real-estate records almost every day in order to keep tabs on the living arrangements of the stars in his book. He also continually adds the addresses of new stars. On the afternoon we met, Gordon was preparing to track down the home of Robert Pastorelli, who had once played the role of Eldin, the live-in housepainter on the sitcom *Murphy Brown*. Pastorelli had killed himself about a month earlier, and had been a suspect in the murder of his girlfriend. The crime had occurred at Pastorelli's home, and this interested Gordon because he planned to create a new section in his book focusing on celebrity murders. "I have a photo of Pastorelli's home from this old *TV Guide* clipping," he said, brandishing a partially torn piece of glossy paper. "So we should be able to find the place."

Without further ado, Gordon and I hopped into his car and headed upward along a road that wound its way into the higher reaches of Beverly Hills. As we drove, he provided a running commentary on the homes we passed. "This house here is one that Madonna bought from Diane Keaton and is now trying to sell for about ten million dollars," he said, pointing at a gigantic Spanish-style hacienda. "Now we are coming up to Angelina

Jolie's house. Angelina and Madonna are the only stars dumb enough to move onto streets that are frequented by the tour buses. Everyone else asks for houses that are off the beaten path."

Gordon proceeded to tell me about the many "survival jobs" he'd had in his professional life. "These were jobs that paid the rent but ate away at your soul, and left you wondering each night, 'Why am I doing this?' And that's the nice thing about what I'm doing now. I look forward to going to work each day. I enjoy driving around Los Angeles and Hollywood, even though it's basically a frivolous thing to do. Bear in mind, I went to college at UCLA, which is just a couple of miles from here, and back then I would have turned up my nose at this kind of stuff." He had initially aspired to write nonfiction books of a more serious nature. In fact, he had spent much of the 1970s researching the shootings at Kent State University, and his findings were published in a book called *Four Dead in Ohio*. "This was during the Vietnam era, and I was interested in the war and what was going on in the world," Gordon said. "It's funny, though, when you get older, you just learn that there is nothing you can do about it—so you just tune it out."

"So you were pretty politically active during the 1960s?" I asked.

"Not really," he replied. "I spent most of the 1960s in the library, which is also where I spent most of the 1970s." He interrupted our conversation to point out a house where the Mamas and the Papas had once lived, before they were evicted for not paying rent. He slowed our car to a crawl so that I could get a good look at the place, and then he hit the accelerator. "These are my escapism years," he told me as the wind fluttered in through the windows. "With this war in Iraq, we might be going down the road to another Vietnam, and I am offering myself— and others—an escape from the harsh day-to-day realities of life." Gordon recalled that during the Watergate hearings many housewives complained that their favorite soap operas were being interrupted by the news coverage. This seemed odd to him at the time, but now it made sense. "People are like that. They like to shut it out. And these are my don't-bother-me-with-anything-important years. I think this is a phase. At some point I would like to do something more substantive again, like a true-crime book."

"Do you think you will?"

"I hope so. The thing is, there is a built-in audience for this celebrity stuff." One indication of this, Gordon insisted, was the fact that unlike *The Ultimate Hollywood Tour Book,* his book on the Kent State shootings sold only several thousand copies. Of course, there are indications more dramatic than this. Every day millions of Americans search for information about the stars. According to the search engine Yahoo!, eight of the ten most popular search terms for 2005 were the names of celebrities, with Britney Spears at the top of the list. "The truth is, many people's lives are empty, and they latch on to these celebrities," Gordon said. "It's easier to talk about celebrities than our own lives, which is another kind of escapism—not from Vietnam or Iraq but from the boredom of one's own life. Celebrities are probably of less interest to people who live exciting, fulfilling lives—people who are involved with their family and community. But how many people do you know who live exciting, fulfilling lives?"

Before I could answer, Gordon pulled his car over to the curb and looked around as if disoriented. "No wonder I'm lost," he muttered. "*There* is Brad Pitt's house, and *there* is Danny DeVito's house." He nodded, smiled, and pulled back onto the road. "I got a little turned around," he told me. "But now I know where I am."

Bill Gordon is not alone in observing that Americans appear to be uninvolved with their families and communities. In 2000 Robert Putnam, of Harvard University, published *Bowling Alone,* in which he argues compellingly that Americans increasingly feel lonely and alienated from one another. In his book Putnam draws heavily on a life-style study from the marketing firm DDB, which is based in Chicago. The latest statistics from DDB, which I obtained for this book, continue to support Putnam's claim. For example, Americans' attendance at club meetings in 2005 was a third of what it had been in 1975. Ties with friends and family are also weakening. In 1980 Americans entertained friends at home sixteen times a year, on average. By 2005 they were doing so fewer than eight times. And the percentage of Americans who said their family "definitely" ate together on a regular basis fell by a third between 1975 and 1999, and continued to fall slightly through 2005. According to DDB, even the average number of picnics Americans make each year has dropped by more than 60 percent in the thirty years since 1975.

There is also evidence that we use celebrities as coping mechanisms when we feel lonely or don't expect to connect with others. In a study conducted by Jean Twenge, of San Diego State University, a group of college students took a personality test and were then randomly divided into three groups. The first, the "future belonging" group, was told that their personality tests foretold a future with a strong network of friends and loved ones. The second, the "future alone" group, was essentially told to expect a life of loneliness and isolation. Members of the third were told that they could expect a life of being accident-prone. After receiving this news, all the subjects were given a choice: they could spend the next few minutes filling out a health questionnaire to receive valuable feedback about their physical health, or they could read *People* or *Entertainment Weekly*. Members of the "future alone" group were more than twice as likely as members of either of the other two groups to choose the magazines.

Twenge's interest in celebrities, and how we use them as coping mechanisms, led her to conduct another study in a similar vein. She asked a group of college students to take the same personality test and then she arbitrarily divided them into two groups; half were told to expect a life of loneliness, and half to expect a life of being accident-prone. Then she divided each group into three subgroups: one was asked to write about a family member, one about a celebrity, and one about the food served at a recent meal. Finally Twenge asked all the subjects to play a game that tested their levels of aggression: they were to blast a human subject with loud noise whenever the subject didn't complete a task quickly enough. Twenge hypothesized that the "future alone" group would be more aggressive, but that the members of its subgroup who had just written about a family member would be calmed by the thought of the strong personal relationships they *did* have within their family. She was right—but members of the "future alone" subgroup who wrote about celebrities were also far less aggressive. Twenge concluded that celebrities, like family members, offer us a means of warding off feelings of loneliness and aggression. This became particularly clear to her, she says, when she read her subjects' essays on celebrities, many of which were written in warm personal tones. "It didn't sound like they were talking about celebrities," she told me. "It sounded like they were talking about their best friends from the third grade."

In my youth, I can remember watching the movie *Risky Business* and thinking that the character played by Tom Cruise would be a great best friend to have. According to the producer, Steve Tisch, this was no accident. Tisch is a tall man with a strong jaw and close-cropped graying hair. His reputation in Hollywood comes from having produced successful movies such as *Forrest Gump, Snatch, American History X,* and *Risky Business.* But perhaps above all, Tisch is known as the producer who discovered Tom Cruise. He says that he and his partner Jon Avnet had spent months looking for an actor to play the lead in *Risky Business.* One day Tom Cruise walked into his office, and almost instantly Tisch knew that he was the one. Tisch insists that the secret to Cruise's appeal is that on top of being a heartthrob, he is almost universally likable: "Unlike many other talented actors who have emerged over the past twenty years, Tom Cruise will get the girl in the audience, but he will also get the husband or the boyfriend, because they want to be his pal. The girls love him, but the guys aren't threatened by him. That's key. Cruise is cool, but not so cool that he would ignore you. He is endearing, charismatic, warm, and funny, without ever being threatening. You would let this guy drive your girlfriend home after school. What it comes down to is that this is a guy who you'd want to bring home and introduce as your new best friend."

Bonnie Fuller, the chief editorial director for American Media Inc., the tabloid conglomerate that publishes the *Star,* the *National Enquirer,* and the *Globe,* says that the real allure of celebrities is not that they replace our friends but that they help us find new ones. "What's going on is that we all have fewer people in common," Fuller told me. "When you're in high school, or at a small college, you know everybody's business and you can follow their romantic goings-on and discuss them with your friends. But when you grow up and you're out in the work world, you don't have that. So celebrities give us a whole world of people in common—people to gossip about at work over the water cooler or at a dinner party."

The psychologist Robin Dunbar notes that the word "gossip" didn't always have tawdry connotations. Dunbar writes, "The term *gossip* itself did not originally have that [negative] meaning. It meant simply the activity that one engaged in with one's 'god-sibs,' one's peer group equivalent of godparents: in other words, those with whom one was especially close." Dunbar believes that language actually evolved in order to facilitate gossip, which played a crucial role in helping early humans to form alliances and groups. Nowadays, says Dunbar, gossip is still important, because it allows us to advertise our "advantages as a friend, ally, or mate."

As Bonnie Fuller sees it, because they facilitate gossip, celebrities are catalysts for bringing us together. This strikes me as true, but only to a point. For example, when we gossip about our friends and acquaintances, we know and can interact with the people involved. So if my friend Cindy's boyfriend dumped her, I could gossip about it, but I could also take Cindy out to dinner, listen to her woes, and give her some advice. If and when the time came, Cindy could do the same for me. Meanwhile, we might learn about each other's lives, help each other cope with a range of emotions, and ultimately develop a deep and lasting connection. In short, our *gossip* might lead us to become *godsibs*. Ideally, this is how relationships—and, in fact, communities—work. But celebrities often distract us from this. So when I bump into my coworkers after hours, instead of talking about *our* marriages, we talk about Brad Pitt's marriage. Our discussions of Brad Pitt may sometimes segue into more meaningful discussions of our own lives, but more often than not they lead to Angelina Jolie, or Jennifer Aniston, or the movies, or practically anything other than ourselves.

Not long after my outing with Bill Gordon in Beverly Hills, I found myself in midtown Manhattan at the weekly editorial meeting for *Us Weekly*. Just before noon about twenty staff members shuffled into a giant glass tank of a room that sat in the middle of a sprawling labyrinth of grayish cubicles. The room's only color came from a large bulletin board, which was wallpapered with the covers of past issues that paired fleshy glam shots of celebrities with pithy headlines reading "How Jen Found Out," "Why Brad Said Goodbye," "J-Lo: I am ready for a baby," "Justin Didn't Cheat on Me," and "Nick & Jessica: Will they split?" These were some of the hottest-selling covers in the country. During the first six months of 2005, newsstand sales of *Us Weekly* rose by 32.6 percent, to 989,011. The big picture looked just as good. Between 1995 and 2005, total circulation was up by 39 percent, hitting an impressive 1.67 million by mid-2005. The boom in sales could be traced back to 2000, when Bonnie Fuller and Janice Min, two of the magazine's top editors, collaborated to redesign the monthly *Us* and turn it into *Us Weekly*. (At the time Fuller was the magazine's editor-in-chief, though she has left since then, and Min now has that job.) The magazine's old template had featured longer celebrity profiles; the new one combined dozens of luscious photos with shorter, punchier articles on a large cast of celebrities who appeared in almost every issue. The formula was a resounding success, and the magazine's staff has been scrambling ever since to keep its pages filled with these sorts of stories.

"Hey, did you see the quote by Gwyneth in *Time* magazine where she dissed Brad for not being more private about his relationships?" Bradley Jacobs, the senior editor in charge of film coverage, asked. The staff members nodded. "Why don't we do a story on everyone who has dissed their exes in public?" he asked. "Because didn't Ben just talk about Jen in *Elle*?"

"Yeah," said one of the twentysomething women at the conference table who were dressed in chic-casual style—jeans, tight tennis shirts, and flip-flops with pedicured toenails. "And I think Nicole talked about Tom in *Vanity Fair* . . ."

"Right, and Britney Murphy dissed Ashton on Leno or Letterman," said another.

"Good," said Jacobs, who was jotting down notes. Clearly a story was coming together. ("This is how we like to do it," he told me later. "We try to take a quote like this and build a two-page feature out of it by providing six or seven other examples.") The same formula was at work again several minutes later, when Michael Steele, the magazine's executive editor, proposed a story about celebrities who had once worked at fastfood restaurants. According to Steele, Brad Pitt had gotten his start at a restaurant on the corner of La Brea and Sunset Boulevards, where he donned a giant chicken costume, waved at traffic, and received jeers from passersby. "They weren't yelling at me," Pitt allegedly insisted. "They were yelling at the damn chicken!" As I soon learned, Madonna had sold glazed edibles at Dunkin' Donuts, Andie MacDowell had shoveled fries at McDonald's, Queen Latifah had slaved away at Burger King, Pink had worked at Wendy's, Jason Lee had pushed Mexican fare at Taco Bell, and Marcia Gay Harden had worked at Howard Johnson's.

During these discussions an attractive woman in her midthirties, with pearl earrings and blazing-white teeth, sat at the head of the table, sipping a cold drink and looking pleased. This was

Janice Min. By her own admission, Min is an unlikely candidate to be running the magazine. "Growing up, I was not one of these girls who hung posters of celebrities on her wall," she later told me. "And I think that *not* growing up as a celebrity addict has been incredibly helpful." Min seems to exude a certain detachment from the subject matter she covers, and she claims that this enables her to focus on what the readers want. "One of the most popular sections of the magazine is the 'Stars—They're Just Like Us!' section," she said. "At its essence, it is this preposterous little photo act showing celebrities shopping for groceries or getting gas or eating a pizza—but it's just incredibly compelling to the reader."

The demystification of movie stars is something that has gradually occurred over the past century. In the very early days of Hollywood not even the names of stars were revealed, and moviegoers had to refer to their favorites rather vaguely, as "the girl with the curls," "the sad-eyed man," or "the fat guy." In *Picture Personalities,* Richard deCordova writes that fans soon began asking theater managers and movie studios for more information about their favorite stars. Sometime around 1909, for example, a teenage fan of the actress Florence Lawrence wrote her a letter (care of her film studio) in which he addressed her as "Dear Stranger" and begged her to reveal her true name. By the 1930s a number of "fanzines" were running long, gushing profiles of celebrities. An issue of *Photoplay* from 1935 described the actress Loretta Young this way: "Loretta Young is a beauty, one of the most ethereally beautiful women in the world. She was born to be loved and cherished and worshipped by men. In other ages, men would have fought for her favor, gladiators would have ridden to death for her glove." By World War II, however, demystification was well under way. In 1940 *Life* magazine ran a feature that showed movie stars living rather modestly. "Their homes, once gaudy and too ornate, are now as sensible and sound in taste as any in the country," the text read. By the 1960s celebrity news magazines had abandoned any remaining reverence for the stars and begun gravitating toward scandalous themes. In 1967, for example, *Movie Mirror* ran an article about Elizabeth Taylor titled "Liz Will Adopt a Negro Baby!" A few years later *Movie Life* ran the headline "Why Shirley Jones's Sex Opinions Broke Up Her Marriage," and *Motion Picture* carried a story titled "Cops Seize Onassis's Dirty Picture Collection." The next big shift came in 1974, when *People* was founded and began publishing articles about celebrities alongside human-interest stories about ordinary people who had experienced tragedy or shown great courage. In effect, *People* continued the process of demystifying the famous by placing everyday Americans alongside Hollywood celebrities in issue after issue. According to Ray Browne, a professor emeritus at Bowling Green University who has been studying celebrity magazines since the 1950s, this ongoing demystification reflects people's desire to feel better about themselves. "Throughout much of history our heroes have been exalted and placed on pedestals," he told me. "We talked about Lord Nelson, or Mr. Grant, or Miss Hepburn. But the trend over the past several decades has been to take celebrities off their pedestals, because by doing this we raise our own sense of self."

According to the editors at *Us Weekly,* the secret to the magazine's success is that they have perfected the art of portraying celebrities as friendly, down-to-earth, neighborly people. The "Stars—They're Just Like Us!" section does this best. Most of these articles have a casual and friendly tone. "We shy away from any story that would make the reader feel creepy and intrusive," Michael Steele explained. "It's one thing to do a cheerful little story about a celebrity couple that goes out for a sushi date, in which we run a picture of them walking out of the restaurant, smiling and holding hands. It's another thing to show them caught during an awkward moment and waving their hands like, *Please don't take my picture!* The reader will be turned off by this. And it's important that our readers not feel as if they're making their favorite stars miserable, because our readers *like* these celebrities."

This made perfect sense to me: if the reader comes to feel that he or she is snooping on private moments, then the chummy, intimate magic the magazine creates is broken. And this may be the real power behind *Us Weekly:* it offers the illusion of friendship. "Our readers feel like Jennifer Aniston is their best friend," Bradley Jacobs said during one of our chats. "There's a reason the magazine is doing better than ever this year. Jen became everyone's best friend in the TV show *Friends,* and then she breaks up with Brad and has this big trauma. Has this raised magazine sales? Absolutely!"

Before leaving *Us Weekly,* I visited Janice Min's office, which had recently been recarpeted and was in a state of disarray—boxes were all over the place, alongside Rolodexes, bottles of Perrier, photos from the most recent MTV Video Music Awards, and an old Kermit the Frog doll sitting next to a Prada suit bag. Min took a seat at her desk, and, as she eased back from the morass of papers on her desk, we started talking about why the magazine's readers were so devoted to celebrities.

"Whether the public has grown delusional or not," Min said, "it seems like they want to feel this connection to the celebs they love, which is why they refer to them on a first-name basis. Jennifer Aniston is now just 'Jen.' Brad Pitt is just 'Brad.' Jennifer Lopez is 'J-Lo.' I always find it funny whenever I'm at a bar or a restaurant and I can hear a group of young women in their twenties, and they just go off on someone—they start talking about Brad and Angelina, and they move seamlessly into a discussion about their own sister or best friend or their job, and then back into a discussion of Brad and Angelina. All of a sudden these celebrities have become a part of their peer group. That distinction between *us* and *them* no longer exists."

On my way out of Min's office someone handed me a stack of back issues. On the subway I began to flip through them. As my train rattled uptown, I noticed an elderly woman engrossed in the current issue of *Us Weekly,* straining her eyes in the flickering light to look at pictures of Brad and Jen. In the coming days I saw dozens of other people reading the magazine, including several teenage girls, a man in a business suit, a hairdresser, and a sleepy-eyed night watchman. As hard as I tried, I couldn't see what they had in common. I doubted that *all* of them were lonely or bored with their lives. Even if they were, it seemed unlikely that this alone explained why they were reading this particular magazine. Clearly other forces had to be at play. And according to Michael Platt, of Duke University, those forces may be best understood by studying the behavior of monkeys.

Platt is a tall, dapper-looking man in his late thirties. His deep-blue eyes, tanned complexion, and silvery goatee give him the air of an art dealer from SoHo. One would never guess that he spends much of his time working with monkeys. Platt's specialty is "decision theory," a field that investigates how ecology, evolution, and neurobiology affect the decision-making process. He studies the behavior of rhesus monkeys, also known as rhesus macaques, which grow to be about two feet in length and thirteen pounds in weight. As it turns out, rhesus monkeys are quite popular in the halls of science. In the 1950s and 1960s NASA launched a number of them into space. Decades later, in 2001, a rhesus monkey named Tetra became the first cloned primate. Platt is interested in how rhesus monkeys think. In 2005 he and his postdoctoral assistant, Robert Deaner, demonstrated for the first time that rhesus monkeys, like humans, value information for its social content. We know that people pay to see pictures of powerful or sexually attractive individuals; according to this study, monkeys expend resources to do the same thing.

I met Platt at his laboratory in Durham, a large, modern building with the warm, ripe smell of a primate house at the zoo, and he gave me a quick tour of the facility. We walked down a long cement corridor and peered into a room containing several caged rhesus monkeys. "You see that guy on the left?" Platt asked, pointing at a monkey that appeared to be jeering at me. "You see how he is staring right at you and showing his teeth like that? That's because he is threatening you." Platt smiled at me half apologetically. "And you see the guy on the right who's smacking his lips at you and pulling his ears back? Well, he is more or less submitting to you."

Like most of the other researchers in his lab, Platt has become adept at reading the gestures and body language of the monkeys in his troop, which allows him to understand the troop's power dynamics. After extensive observation he concluded that two of the monkeys, Sherwood and Wolfgang, were the toughest and fiercest in the troop, because all the other monkeys tended to defer to them by giving them submissive gestures. Once this was determined, Platt wanted to know if the subordinate monkeys would give up food in order to look at pictures of Sherwood and Wolfgang.

Platt eventually led me down to the testing area—a small, barren cinder-block room equipped with several computers and a mini-fridge holding enough Juicy Juice to feed a large class of screaming kindergarteners. Juicy Juice played a crucial role in Platt's experiment. "We put the monkeys in one of these so-called monkey chairs," he said, wheeling out a large plastic device that looked like a giant highchair. "Then we position them in front of a computer screen that flashes various images. We can tell what the monkeys are looking at, because we have implanted tiny electronic devices over their eyes. Depending on where they look, we reward them by squirting various amounts of Juicy Juice into their mouths."

The experiment presented the monkeys with a series of choices. In each case two images would flash on the screen at the same time: a blank gray square and a digital photo of a monkey from the troop. If they looked at the gray square, they got the same amount of Juicy Juice every time. But if they looked at the monkey, the payment varied. There were four basic types of photos: [1] frontal shots of dominant males, [2] frontal shots of subordinate males, [3] frontal shots of females, and [4] close-up shots of females' hindquarters. Platt discovered that the monkeys were willing to "pay" (give up Juicy Juice) to stare at females' hindquarters or at dominant males. But they had to "be paid" (get extra Juicy Juice) to stare at frontal photos of females or subordinate males.

Within the realm of neuroscience this study was groundbreaking. Prior to 2005, when it was published, no one had attempted to study how animals value the opportunity to acquire information, especially social information—partly because no one had figured out how to measure this. Platt gave his monkeys a quantifiable currency (i.e., Juicy Juice), and the monkeys went on to make some interesting choices. The question became, What motivated these choices?

There are good evolutionary explanations for why Platt's monkeys acted as they did. Male monkeys in the wild enhance their chances of reproducing by studying females' hindquarters to discern which of the females in their troop are most aroused and interested in mating. They also keep a close eye on what the dominant males are doing, in order to avoid trouble—just as a kid nervously keeps an eye on a bully who enters the schoolyard. The monkeys may also watch a dominant male in hopes of finding a window of opportunity—when he is asleep, not paying attention, or simply absent—that allows them to sneak off and mate with one of the females. Over time those monkeys who were more adept at gathering information about dominant males and sexually receptive females may well have had better luck at surviving and reproducing.

The same thing may apply to humans. It is quite possible that our modern-day desire to keep tabs on the powerful and the sexy, à la *Us Weekly,* stems from our ancient past. In prehistoric times a man would want to gather as much information as he could about his group's leader: how he was feeling, what he liked to eat, which females he favored, whether he had been hunting, if he'd been injured, where he liked to rest, when he usually went to sleep, and how long he slept. All this information would have helped him forge alliances, or plot a coup, or make plans to have sex covertly with one of the leader's women. A socially astute early man with a keen eye for gathering information on the powerful was probably far more likely to survive and reproduce—especially if he also looked out for the most fertile and sexually receptive females. Over time, this sort of natural selection may have favored behavior similar to celebrity-watching.

"In our society this ancient behavioral adaptation may now just be going wild," Platt suggests. "The media has simply expanded our social group to include practically everyone on the planet, so we get stuck gazing at powerful celebrities we don't even know." We are hard-wired to gather all this social information about powerful people, he concludes, but much of what we gather in the media is useless.

Yet if humans are predisposed to watch powerful people, why aren't they fixating on C-SPAN2 and its coverage of the House Armed Services Committee? A few explanations are possible. The first is that entertainment celebrities, unlike politicians, usually strive to maintain an image that is both powerful and sexy. When Angelina Jolie arrives at the Oscars, she enjoys all the trappings of power—a long limousine, security guards, a roped-off entranceway, a regal red carpet—but she also wears a low-cut evening gown and exudes sexuality. So TV viewers are seeing the equivalent of dominant-male photos and female-hindquarters photos in one irresistible package. Women probably experience something similar when Brad Pitt arrives in his limo.

Another explanation is simply that A-list celebrities dramatically radiate power in a way that very few politicians do. We read that Tom Cruise earned $70 million for a single movie, that Sharon Stone owns a $22,000 crocodile-skin coat, that presenters at the Oscars got gift baskets worth more than $30,000, and that Russell Crowe threw a ceramic vase at a hotel concierge who wasn't sufficiently accommodating. By contrast, it's doubtful that any politician could exhibit such ostentatious and swaggering behavior, because it would offend our democratic sensibilities. Even the wealthiest and most headstrong politicians must at least feign being humble, polite, and down-to-earth in order to win over their constituents. It's hard to imagine a U.S. senator who could appear on *The Oprah Winfrey Show* and jump up and down on a couch with relative impunity, as Tom Cruise once did.

In some ways, the demeanor of some modern-day celebrities

is reminiscent of behavior that the primatologist Frans de Waal observed in chimps at the Arnhem Zoo, in the Netherlands. De Waal noted that one of the dominant chimps, Yeroen, liked to stage veritable rock concerts during which he would demand the attention of all the other chimps by standing on a large yellow drum and jumping wildly until "the whole building boomed with the sound of his drumming." If a dominant chimp like Yeroen didn't receive sufficient attention and respect, de Waal writes in *Chimpanzee Politics,* he would sometimes go into a rage: "With an unerring sense of drama he would let himself drop out of a tree like a rotten apple and roll around on the ground screaming and kicking."

Platt says this may be precisely the sort of "dominant" behavior that our brains have evolved to recognize as being noteworthy: "When we see celebrities strutting about, exhibiting these bold and inflated patterns of behavior, presumably our brains are recognizing this behavior and telling us, *This is a person you need to pay attention to in order to survive and reproduce.* Whereas when we see a senator from South Dakota, we immediately assume that he is unimportant and ignore him."

Of course, if you ask people why they like to look at pictures of Brad Pitt or Angelina Jolie, they may say—if they're not too embarrassed to admit it—that it's simply enjoyable. According to evolutionary psychologists, that feeling is the direct result of natural selection, because those people who "enjoyed" such observation were more likely to survive and reproduce. Douglas Kenrick, an evolutionary psychologist at Arizona State University who studies popular culture, likes to make this point with ice cream. According to Kenrick, when we eat a bowl of Ben & Jerry's, we aren't usually thinking about the evolutionary backstory of *why* it tastes so delicious. Yet the fact is that throughout much of human history people were practically starving, and needed to eat fats and sugars in order to survive. Taste buds that favored rich foods like Ben & Jerry's were actually advantageous. Hollywood celebrities are a lot like Ben & Jerry's, Kenrick says, because they, too, trigger ancient evolutionary mechanisms: "Historically, those humans who paid attention to status and power did better. The same is true of those who paid attention to fertile women who looked like they might be interested in sex." The way Kenrick sees things, it makes perfect evolutionary sense that both Ben & Jerry's and Angelina Jolie are irresistible.

Toward the end of my time at Duke, I followed Platt back to his office, which was filled with books and ape paraphernalia, including a large bust of a gorilla that Platt had had since high school and a framed photo of Nim Chimpsky, a legendary chimp who knew how to use sign language. I asked Platt whether, from an evolutionary perspective, there was anything to be gained by following the lives of celebrities.

"Yes," he said. "Can you imagine someone who is a shut-in, who doesn't know anything about celebrities? It's quite possible that they would fail to integrate into society, appear strange, get no dates, and ultimately not reproduce. So theoretically, those who tune in to celebrities may end up with an advantage in the reproductive race." Platt paused and then offered a sheepish smile. "Makes sense, doesn't it?"

8

A Choice of Worship: Rod *vs.* God

MARCY BRAUNSTEIN, of Pittsburgh, Pennsylvania, has devoted much of her life to Rod Stewart—following him around the world to attend his concerts, making "pilgrimages" to his home in Hollywood and his birthplace in England, and even building a shrine, or "Rod Room," in her house. Braunstein was therefore quite dismayed when she visited Los Angeles and discovered that Stewart had no star on the Hollywood Walk of Fame—that legendary stretch of sidewalk where pink stars etched with celebrities' names are embedded in the concrete.

Since the late 1950s, when the Walk of Fame was created, more than 2,000 stars have been awarded to movie and TV actors and an assortment of other celebrities, including Thomas Edison (who is credited with inventing motion pictures), Big Bird, Pee Wee Herman, and two dogs: Lassie and Rin Tin Tin. For many devoted fans, the Walk of Fame is holy ground. Indeed, on any given day, fans are paying homage to their favorite celebrities by laying flowers on the concrete or simply bending down to touch the ground. The star belonging to Julio Iglesias is always in pristine condition, for example, because a devoted band of elderly women comes to scrub and polish it once a month.

Clearly Rod Stewart—a Grammy-winning musician who is still one of the best-selling recording artists in America—has earned a place on the Walk of Fame. But as Marcy Braunstein discovered, no one had ever bothered to nominate him. Upon making this discovery, she quickly filled out a nomination form and began raising money on the Internet from other Stewart fans to cover the induction fee of $15,000.

The induction process for the Walk of Fame is a Byzantine affair that requires approval from a series of agencies, including the Hollywood Chamber of Commerce, the Department of Public Works for the City of Los Angeles, the Los Angeles City Council, and the Office of the (honorary) Mayor of Hollywood—an eighty-two-year-old former talk-show host named Johnny Grant. According to Mayor Grant, who presides over the entire process, he is constantly approached by would-be inductees and their friends. "I was at a funeral the other day, and someone was telling me about a candidate who 'deserved' to be on the Walk of Fame," Grant told me. "And I told 'em, 'I think this is very inappropriate!'" Once the application process is under way, things can turn contentious, as officials bicker over who is or isn't a bona fide celebrity. "We've had some knock-down, drag-out fights," Grant said. "We've got one guy on the chamber committee who says for every nomination, 'Why would you want to give that asshole a star?'"

Fortunately for Braunstein and Stewart, his nomination sailed through without complications. It was approved in June of 2005, just weeks after it had been submitted. Braunstein immediately started planning her trip to Los Angeles for the award ceremony, where, as Stewart's official nominator, she would help present him with his star.

I visited Braunstein several weeks before her trip to Los Angeles. When I arrived at her small, blue, aluminum-sided house situated on the edge of a steep bluff in a middle-class suburb of Pittsburgh, she answered the door wearing jeans and a Rod Stewart T-shirt. Braunstein was a plump, fifty-two-year-old woman with blond hair, rosy cheeks, and glossy magenta fingernails. On her feet, she wore faux leopard-skin slippers. The slippers, she explained, were a tribute to Stewart.

"I've been into Rod for over twenty years," she said, escorting me into the kitchen and offering me a tall glass of iced tea. "The first time I heard him was back in 1972, and I just fell in love with him. It is hard to put into words exactly why. I guess it's the whole package—the hair, the raspy tenor of the voice, the high cheekbones—it just drives me crazy." She sipped her iced tea and then added with a nervous laugh, "Who would have known that twenty-five or thirty years later I would still be running around the country going to Rod concerts? Back then this notion would have seemed crazy to me, because I was in college and I was looking for bigger and better things."

Since then Braunstein had finished school, gotten married, landed a job as an administrator at a local blood bank, and gradually become more and more devoted to Stewart. On a few occasions she had a chance to meet him in person—albeit briefly—by waiting for him in the lobby of his hotel or by going to one of his promotional events. Once she even had a brief conversation with him backstage. At this point, Braunstein said, Stewart did seem to recognize her, but they weren't exactly on a first-name basis.

"Hey," she said with a sudden burst of enthusiasm. "Do you want to see my Rod Room?"

As we took a narrow flight of carpeted stairs to the second floor, Braunstein said, "You know, I like to joke that if my husband and I ever had kids, my Rod Room would be a nursery. But it's not. In any case, everyone has to have their baby—everybody has to have their thing. And mine happens to be Rod Stewart."

At the top of the stairs, we made a hard left and stopped for a moment in front of a bedroom door. "My father thinks I should put holy water here so you can dip your fingers and shake them before entering," she said. "And just so you know, sometimes people get a little overwhelmed." That said, she led the way into the room, which was crammed floor to ceiling with more artifacts and memorabilia than one might expect to find in the presidential library of a lesser-known American president. There were, among many other things, roughly twenty framed and autographed photos of Stewart (many of which included the pen he had used), every album he ever recorded, a dozen different Rod Stewart coffee mugs, a copy of Braunstein's license plate, which read ROD FAN, a framed dress shirt Stewart once wore, and a glass he once sipped from on *Oprah*. Based on her experiences of buying and selling Rod artifacts on eBay, Braunstein estimated that her collection was worth about $25,000—roughly half her annual salary.

"When I first started going on eBay," she said, "if there was some collectible, or rare album, or some magazine cover that I didn't have, there would be no limit to what I would pay for it. But now if there's something I want, I'll make myself wait a couple of days. When you are so crazy and passionate about someone, the way I am with Rod, you simply want *everything* that has to do with them. If they are on TV, for example, you want to make sure you make a tape of it. And if, heaven forbid, I did not set the VCR properly—which has happened a couple of times—I just go crazy afterward, and then I have to get a copy of the tape. I've called out to Los Angeles and paid a hundred dollars just to get a copy of a Jay Leno episode that I missed." The most trying moments, she said, occurred when Stewart was taking time off. "When he is *not* on tour, I'll chat online with other Rod fans and we'll say that we are going through 'Rod withdrawal,' or we need a 'Rod fix.' Now it looks like Rod and his fiancée, Penny Lancaster, will soon be having a baby, and Rod has said he probably won't go on tour in 2006. And in my mind I'm thinking, *Well, I'm going to see him in October, at the Walk of Fame event, so that should get me through.*"

For a while we sat in silence and took in the panorama of the room. The effect was somewhat dizzying: my eyes began to glaze over as I looked at the endlessly repeated features of Rod Stewart—the slightly crooked nose, the naughty smile, the spiky haircut, the rosy cheeks, and the abundance of leopard-skin clothing—which soon seemed to intermix like fragments in a whirling kaleidoscope.

"There is one thing we haven't talked about," Braunstein said finally. "And we should probably discuss it before my husband, Dave, gets home." I found this sudden proclamation puzzling, but I simply nodded my head, and waited for Marcy to continue. "I believe in the sanctity of marriage," she said. "I'm very in love with my husband, and I know in my heart of hearts that I couldn't leave him. But sometimes people ask me, 'What would you do if Rod came by one day and said, 'Hey, Marcy, let's go!' Of course, I know that's not even a remotely likely scenario. But it certainly would be a dilemma."

Braunstein's husband, Dave Jones, returned home moments later, almost on cue. He was a tall, powerfully built African American man dressed in a beige jogging suit and sneakers. His tightly cropped hair and meticulously trimmed mustache were dark gray. Over a late lunch in the kitchen I asked him what he thought of his wife's passion for Rod Stewart.

"She doesn't drink, and she doesn't smoke, so this is literally the only enjoyment she actually has," he replied. "But I'm going to be honest: there is no way I could put my foot down, because she would never listen anyway. And if I tried, it would be like 'You can go, because Rod is staying.'" Jones said that over the years he had resigned himself to becoming a Rod Stewart fan too. He still preferred jazz, but he was able to enjoy a good Rod Stewart concert—even though he was usually the only black man in the audience. When I asked him what this was like, he smiled and said, "It feels powerful. Everyone thinks I am someone. Everyone wants to know who I am and whether I'm a member of the band." Another perk of being a Stewart fan was that he had become friendly with the singer's statuesque blond fiancée, Penny Lancaster. Apparently Lancaster often came out into the audience at concerts and said hello to regulars like Jones and Braunstein. The couple had enjoyed far more contact with her than with Stewart. "Penny hugs me at almost every show," Jones said. "So literally Marcy can do what she likes because she has Rod, and as long as I can be around Penny, I don't care."

"Penny just gravitates toward Dave," Braunstein said proudly, putting a hand on her husband's shoulder. "Dave loves it. And besides, I think that if Dave hadn't become a Rod fan—and if I had continued to be this interested in Rod—it might have caused problems in our marriage."

As the afternoon wore on, eventually the conversation turned to Braunstein's niece, Mary Grace, who was attending the Moody Bible Institute, in Chicago. During a visit to Pittsburgh when Mary Grace was in her early teens, she once wandered into the Rod Room and expressed her concern. "You know," she told her aunt, "this could be considered idol worshiping." Braunstein, who attends church regularly and considers herself a devout Christian, assured her niece that she had the wrong impression. But privately she was slightly rattled.

"This is something I struggle with," she told me. "I wish that I were as passionate about Jesus—and the life of Jesus and everything that Jesus said when he was on this earth—as I am about Rod. I do worry about that. I worry that I'm worshiping the celebrity of Rod. And I have to ask myself, Would I really travel across the country to attend a rally for Jesus, like I'm doing for this Walk of Fame event with Rod? I don't know.

"I remember when we made our trip to England in 1995 and we visited High Gate, where Rod grew up. What I remember about that visit—and I know this will sound funny—is that I really felt like I was walking on holy ground. I felt like I was walking where someone great had walked. I know how that sounds. And if I went to the Holy Land, and I walked where Christ walked, I would probably feel the same way."

"You see what I have to go through?" Jones said with a shake of his head.

As it turns out, Braunstein is not alone in feeling this way. Despite the apparent rise in prominence of evangelical Christianity within mainstream culture, the fact of the matter is that more and more Americans claim to feel unfulfilled by religion. Since the early 1950s, the Gallup Organization has been conducting polls that gauge how Americans feel about their religions. In 1952, 75 percent of Americans said that religion was "very important" to them; by 2005 that number had dropped to 55 percent. More dramatic than this is that in 1957 only 14 percent of Americans said religion was losing its influence on their lives, and by 2005 that number had risen to 46 percent. The most telling statistics may be those indicating that Americans increasingly feel that religion has little bearing on their lives. In 1957 Gallup began asking respondents, "Do you believe that religion can answer all or most of today's problems, or that religion is largely old-fashioned and out of date?" Those who said religion can answer today's problems dropped from 82 percent in 1957 to 58 percent in 2005. Meanwhile, those who said it was out of date rose from 7 percent to 23 percent over the same time period.

According to Michael Jindra, of Spring Arbor University, in Michigan, who studies how religion and pop culture interact, institutionalized religion may be on the decline, but our thirst for spirituality is not. "Two of the basic things that we need in life, spirituality and connection with others, are traditionally provided for by organized religion," Jindra told me. "We as human beings look for these things, and we form communities around them. So if we're not getting these needs met in one place, we will inevitably look for them somewhere else." That somewhere else, he insists, is increasingly American pop culture.

In the mid-1990s Jindra wrote a paper in which he considered whether die-hard *Star Trek* fans have used the television series and movies to form a new quasi-religion. He describes a *Star Trek* convention at which Trekkies chanted together in a room devoted to prayer, dubbed the Temple of Trek. One of those in attendance was a woman with a newborn baby, which she offered up at one point for "baptism." Another fan told Jindra that she liked to visit the *Star Trek* exhibit at Universal Studios in Los Angeles. "We pilgrimage out there," she said. "That's our Mecca." Jindra concludes that although *Star Trek* fandom "does not seem to fit the more restrictive, substantive definition of religion that posits belief in a deity or in the supernatural," it does have many trappings of organized religion, including a central organization, a recruitment system, and a "canon" of stories or parables.

Jindra believes that pop-culture fans—whether they are Trekkies, *Seinfeld* devotees, or Rod Stewart followers—often seek out experiences that are religious in nature, or attempt to enter "alternate universes." "In the case of *Star Trek,* fans often literally want to step into the universe that Captain Picard and his crew are exploring," he told me. "But fans in general, I believe, often want to enter the 'world' or 'universe' of their favorite celebrity. They do this by watching TV shows or listening to music, of course, but that's just the start. They also enter this universe by collecting paraphernalia, building shrines, and making pilgrimages." These activities give fans a sense of spirituality that is engaging, hands-on, and immediate. According to Jindra, this is especially true when celebrities are involved. "Celebrities lend their own personal charisma to all of this," he says, "and ultimately, traditional religions often find it difficult to compete."

A few research psychologists have looked into the relationship between religiosity and celebrity worship. In 2001 John Maltby, of the University of Leicester, in England, and Lynn McCutcheon, of the DeVry Institute of Technology, in Orlando, conducted a study in which 307 British participants were asked questions that gauged their attitudes toward religion and toward their favorite celebrities. The questions about religion were taken from the Multidimensional Quest Orientation Scale, and asked subjects to rate the veracity of statements such as "I consistently explore issues that will deepen my religious faith" and "I have spent more time compared with most people I know investigating the foundations of my religious faith." The questions about celebrity were taken from the Celebrity Attitude Scale; they asked subjects to rate statements such as "I am obsessed by details of my favorite celebrity's life" and "I would gladly die in order to save the life of my favorite celebrity."

Maltby and McCutcheon found that "as religiosity increases for both men and women the tendency to 'worship' celebrities decreases." This seems to suggest that religiosity and celebrity-worship are mutually exclusive activities—or competing "faiths." But Maltby and McCutcheon also found a distinct subgroup of dual worshipers who scored high on both scales. They concluded, "Many religious people apparently ignore the religious teaching that 'Thou shalt worship no other gods,' or fail to connect it to their 'worship' of celebrities."

Marcy Braunstein appeared to be one of these dual worshipers. This made me wonder whether her two "faiths" were serving separate emotional and spiritual needs. In short, did Rod Stewart offer something that God did not, and vice versa?

The following day, at Braunstein's invitation, I returned to the North Hills of Pittsburgh and joined her, her husband, and their pastor for a more in-depth discussion of celebrity worship. Tim Springs, known as "Pastor Tim" to his congregants at North Hills Community Baptist Church, was a tall man with gray hair and lanky limbs that sprawled across the couch in Braunstein's living room. He listened carefully as Braunstein recounted much of our previous conversation. "I guess my greatest fear," she concluded, "is that someday I'll realize that I could have done something much better with the time, money, enthusiasm, and emotional commitment that I have given to Rod Stewart."

"Well, I don't see this as being overly harmful, as long as it's kept in perspective," Springs said finally. He noted that many people in Pittsburgh were similarly zealous about the Steelers, and he had no problem with this for the most part. As he saw it, people "just want to be a part of something that is larger than them." Sometimes, however, their passion seemed to evolve into what he described as a "sickness"—especially when they felt either happy or depressed based on how the team fared. "I guess that bothers me," Springs said. "Nine years ago I went through my second bout of severe depression, and one of the things I noticed after that was that I couldn't watch the Steelers anymore, because I got too involved. So now I will watch college football instead. But if my wife says 'Let's go for a walk,' then I'll turn it off."

"Hmm," Braunstein said with a slightly worried look. "Now, if I were watching something on TV with Rod Stewart—something live that I hadn't seen before—and Dave wanted to go for a walk . . ."

"Forget it!" Jones interjected.

"Yeah," she confessed. "I really couldn't."

"Do you ever wonder what Rod would make of all this?" Springs asked.

"People have asked me if I think Rod Stewart would perceive me as a stalker," she replied. "But I would never do anything inappropriate."

"What would be inappropriate?" Springs asked. "If you saw him go into hotel room number twelve, would you go up to that room and knock on the door?"

"Well, of course I would," Braunstein replied, banging a fist on the coffee table. "If I knew where he was staying, and he was accessible to me, of course I would—but I wouldn't break into his room."

"So just tell them to keep his door locked," Springs said with a chuckle.

For several seconds an awkward silence enveloped the room.

Braunstein finally turned to her pastor to make a distinction about her feelings toward God and Rod. She truly "worshiped" God, she said, because he was all-knowing, all-loving, and perfect. She even reserved the word "awesome" solely for God. "Now, if you ask me do I worship Rod Stewart . . ."

Jones snorted.

"I am aware of all of Rod's imperfections," Braunstein declared somewhat defensively. "He has a child in England that he doesn't claim. He has botched up marriages. He has broken hearts. He proposed to Penny Lancaster when he's legally still married to Rachel Hunter. I don't look at him and think he is perfect. I guess Rod just makes me feel important. Like when he acknowledges me at a concert, or I get a picture with him. On the other hand, if I'm trying to give him flowers at a concert and he doesn't take them from me, or he takes them from someone else, I'm *crushed*. Because I'm looking to be acknowledged, and when I'm not, I take it personally." She went on to explain that she had no such extreme ups and downs with God. It was steadier all around. "When I first came to Christ, back in 1992,

I felt inner peace. I realize that God loves me just the way I am. Whereas Rod wouldn't. Rod loves tall blondes."

Several weeks later, on the eve of Rod Stewart's induction into the Walk of Fame, Braunstein, Jones, and about a dozen other fans gathered at the Roosevelt Hotel in Hollywood. The hotel, which was built in the 1920s, is a throwback to the Golden Age of Hollywood. Its two-story Spanish-Moorish colonial lobby is framed by hand-painted wooden ceiling beams and leaded-glass windows that cast a murky light on stone floor tiles and gurgling fountains.

Most of the fans were women, with the notable exception of a Rod Stewart impersonator dressed in a leopard-skin jacket and snakeskin pants, who introduced himself to me as "Rod." He added that I could call him "Mini-Rod," so as to prevent any confusion when we were discussing the real Rod. I asked how often he dressed like this, and he replied, "I'll wear this get-up to Home Depot. I have no problem wearing snakeskin pants in public. Most people are shocked and surprised that I can pull it off, but that is why Rod and I have so much in common—we don't care what other people think."

His wife, Diana Graham, added, "When we're out, sometimes people mistake him for the real Rod. It's pretty cool."

The fans were ebullient. They had come from all across the country not only to witness the big event but also to enjoy a spirited reunion with one another. "It's not just seeing Rod Stewart that's fun," said Manny Allbeury, a sixty-year-old British man with gray hair and a heavy Cockney accent. "It's also meeting all these stupid people. We've traveled all over Europe and North America, and we know all the other Rod Stewart idiots. We were just in Germany, and a fellow Rod Stewart idiot over there picked us up at the airport." Allbeury observed that it was now easier than ever for Stewart fans to stay in touch, because of the Internet.

This, in fact, was how Braunstein had organized tonight's gathering—she had put an announcement on three separate Yahoo! message boards, and a band of fans had simply shown up.

According to Linda Kay, a former president of the National Association of Fan Clubs, the Internet has redefined the landscape of fandom. Since the early 1960s the NAFC has been a means for the presidents of some 500 fan clubs to share information about how best to manage and expand their operations. The NAFC's membership encompasses clubs dedicated to an entire gamut of entertainers, including Michael J. Fox, Mel Gibson, Patrick Swayze, Laurel and Hardy, Elvis, several Elvis impersonators, and a performing cat named Princess Kitty. For many years Kay ran the NAFC entirely by herself. In 2002 she decided that she needed a break, so she officially disbanded the organization, though she still maintains its Web site and occasionally advises fan-club presidents. Kay is a forty-one-year-old Web designer from Oceanside, California, who first got serious about fandom when she started a fan club for the band Men at Work, in the early 1980s. In the early 1990s she founded another club, for the movie *Bill and Ted's Excellent Adventure.*

"Back then it was really hard to get members, because it was all word-of-mouth," Kay told me. "But once the Internet came along, suddenly way more people started participating in fan clubs. It's funny, because in the old days joining a fan club was a very geeky and obscure thing to do. Now it's so trendy. Message boards and chat rooms make it so much easier for fans to communicate and form a community, and it opens the clubs to people who *never* in a million years would have done it before." Before the advent of the Internet, Kay says, the fan club for *Bill and Ted's Excellent Adventure* had only 150 members. There is no official membership count nowadays, but the club's Web site, which Kay manages, receives dozens of e-mails each week and roughly 200,000 visits a year. "And this is all for a movie that came out in 1989," she says. "It's really pretty wild."

After chatting for a while with Manny Allbeury, I asked why he and some of his fellow fans described themselves as "idiots."

"Because we are bloody nuts!" he replied. "Who would follow a guy around the whole bloody world? Do you know how much money this costs? Thousands! But that's the way we entertain ourselves. My wife and I don't drink anymore, and we haven't got a mortgage anymore."

"When it comes to Rod Stewart, there are no limits," said his wife, Jean. She pulled out a picture of herself on a stage with Stewart, in which she appeared to be either laughing or crying hysterically.

"What, exactly, is going through your mind here?" I asked.

"She's thinking, *I am going to piss my pants!*" her husband said.

"I'm just feeling excitement," Jean said with a nervous laugh. "It's hard to explain the whole feeling—euphoria, I guess."

As I moved in and out of various conversations among the fans, one of the main topics was the rumor that Stewart was on the verge of taking a year off from touring. A forty-six-year-old woman named Nancy Ortega told me that such a thing would be devastating to her. "That is what we call a serious Rod dry spell," she said. "Because I need my Rod fixes. I'll be driving down the street and I need the fix, so I just pull out one of my thirty-five CDs, and as soon as I play a song, I just feel better. But this is better than having an addiction to other things, isn't it?"

Of all the fans in the lobby that night, none was more visibly excited than Marcy Braunstein. "I get to make a short speech tomorrow at the event," she told me giddily. "I know I'll cry. This will be very emotional. And it'll probably take me weeks to get over this trip. I'd say that this is going to be a big Rod fix— possibly the biggest of all time."

Late in the evening, as the fans' reunion came to an end, Braunstein quietly announced that she and Jones would soon be making a pilgrimage to Stewart's mansion with the Allbeurys. This came as no surprise to me. Many of the others had already told me stories about their visits to Stewart's home. Some simply drove through his neighborhood, some waited for him near his driveway, and others would climb a bluff alongside Denzel Washington's nearby home to get a nice view of Stewart's property. The most remarkable of these stories came from Mini-Rod. "One time I went up to Rod's house to drop off a birthday present for him," he told me. "I was wearing my full Rod uniform, and I had my shades on, so when I pull up to the front gate, the security guard says, 'Hi, Mr. Stewart, are you just going up to the house to drop a few things off?' And I just say, 'Yeah.' Then the gates opened, and I was like, *I'm not worthy.*" Mini-Rod drove around the estate for a while before dropping his birthday present off at the front door, and then he left. He had done this a few times, he told me, but he tried to be discreet about it. "I don't want too many people to know about this. It's a security issue, and there are some real weirdoes out there."

An hour or so later the four fans and I were cruising through the Hollywood Hills in a rental car, looking for Stewart's home. The goal of our pilgrimage was unclear: Jones insisted we were simply doing a drive-by; Braunstein, not surprisingly, was intent on getting out of the car. There was some confusion about the exact location of the house, because Stewart had recently moved. We repeatedly got lost as we wandered along a network of serpentine roads offering spectacular views of the glowing grid of streets below. Jones repeatedly shook his head in disapproval. This was just one of many pilgrimages he had been dragged on. Back in Pittsburgh he had recited a long list of others, such as when his wife had staked out Stewart's floor at the Ritz-Carlton, or had insisted on visiting his penthouse suite at the Taj Mahal. Jones always reluctantly tagged along as her wingman, but tonight he seemed downright bitter. "I just wanted to stay at the hotel tonight," he said. "But she said I had to go."

Eventually we found the entrance to the gated community where Stewart lived. Almost immediately a security guard emerged with a flashlight and motioned for us to keep moving.

"That's it," Jones said. "Let's get out of here."

Braunstein shook her head. She wanted a picture, she said.

For the first time, I saw Jones begin to get angry. "When a security guard tells you to move along, you get your ass out of there!" he yelled.

"This is America!" his wife retorted. "We are allowed to do this." She handed me her digital camera and asked me to snap a photo of the guardhouse. Under pressure I agreed. The camera flashed, and the next thing I knew I heard the wail of police sirens approaching.

"Oh, shit!" said Jones.

For several long moments we sat in tense anticipation of the crisis that was about to ensue. Allbeury laughed nervously. Jones cursed and continued to shake his head. Braunstein said how embarrassed she would be if Stewart found out. And I began envisioning a night in the slammer with nothing but talk of Rod Stewart to sustain me. In the next instant, however, two police cars whizzed past, and we all breathed a sigh of relief.

"So," Allbeury said with a smile. "Now do you see why I call us a bunch of idiots?"

The induction ceremony got going the following morning at around 10:30. Several hundred people, including a great many paparazzi, arrived at the corner of Hollywood Boulevard and Highland Avenue to gather around the bit of sidewalk that now contained Rod Stewart's star. The scene was a madhouse of cameramen and sound engineers, food vendors, teenage Rollerbladers, crisply suited entertainment executives, homeless men in camouflage gear, Japanese tourists, and more than one Rod Stewart impersonator.

Set back from the crowd of onlookers was Mayor Johnny Grant, a dapper, gray-haired man in a pinstripe suit, who sat in a rickety folding chair and leaned forward onto an old black cane. Although he exuded a regal air, Grant has little real authority. His title as mayor is strictly honorary, but not everyone realizes this. He likes to tell the story of a woman who called him up to complain about a large pothole on a back street somewhere in Hollywood. "She told me that she would never vote for me again," Grant told me with a chuckle.

"I consider myself a showman, a hype man, a guy who brings in the tourists," he continued with a flourish of his cane. "After all, the Walk of Fame is not a Nobel Peace Prize ceremony. It's a tourist attraction! In truth, there are few awards that aren't hinged on commercialism. The Oscars and the Grammys are all gimmicks! And while the Walk of Fame might just be a gimmick too—it's certainly no Pulitzer Prize—I've never once seen a dry eye when I've unveiled a new star and said, 'We welcome you to the Walk of Fame!'"

Marcy Braunstein arrived soon after this. She looked nervous almost to the point of being ill. Introducing herself to the mayor, she thanked him profusely for allowing her to participate in the ceremony, and then told him at length about her Rod Room. Grant nodded politely.

"That's nuts!" he said to me after Braunstein had walked away. "But thank God for fans like that who keep the business going."

Although Grant could not remember my name (he kept calling me "Jackson"), he invited me to stick with him during the award ceremony. "Just tell 'em you're my bodyguard," he said.

We made our way to a makeshift stage that stood directly in front of Rod Stewart's gleaming new star. At eleven o'clock sharp Stewart showed up, stepping out of a limo with four of his children and his very pregnant fiancée. He wore white pants, a blue blazer, an orange tie, and his trademark mane of spiky blond hair. The crowd roared with glee, the cameras flashed, and Marcy Braunstein's eyes misted with tears. "I can't believe this is finally happening," she whispered to me. "He's finally going to get his star."

Grant escorted Stewart and Braunstein onto the stage, where he made a speech about the singer's accomplishments, struggling to be heard over the chatter of the crowd. At one point the paparazzi were clamoring so loudly for Stewart's attention that Grant finally yelled, "Enough! You just blew out my hearing aid, so shut up, for Christ's sake!"

After his speech Grant announced that one of Stewart's biggest fans—the woman who had actually nominated him for the Walk of Fame—would now offer some words. Braunstein shakily made her way to the front of the stage, and as she walked past Stewart, their eyes met. Stewart flashed a thousand-watt smile, casually put his arm around her shoulders, and gave her a quick peck on the cheek. He might as well have hit her over the head with a heavy club. She looked stunned. Somehow she maintained her composure and continued toward the microphone. "Rod, my dear," she said, "I think over the years you have seen me hold up a sign at your concert that says 'Lost in you since '72.' And I am here to tell you that you have been singing to my heart since 1972."

Grant edged toward the microphone. Politely but firmly he interjected, "Okay, you got your kiss!"

Braunstein didn't budge. "There are many, many fans who wanted to wish you well today, and most of them are right there," she continued. "And we just want to thank you for everything that you have given us. And, you know, there is just one thing that fans around the world ask: 'Does Rod know what he means to us?' And we hope that he does."

"Thank you!" Grant boomed, and her speech was over.

Next Stewart made a very brief speech in which he thanked his family, his manager, his record label, and all his fans. Then he made his way off the stage and onto the sidewalk, where he posed for photographs alongside his star. The paparazzi immediately began yelling orders at him.

"Put your hand on the star!"

"Put your foot on the star!"

"Dance for us!"

"Kneel down!"

The voices degenerated into a cacophony of wild barks. Soon fans joined the fray, desperately calling for Stewart to autograph some piece of memorabilia. Before long, even casual passersby began stopping to get a closer look, and as they did, a giant, pulsing mob began to form. "Who is at the center of all this?" asked a man who pressed close to me. His wife, who was just a step behind him, was trying to hold him back. I considered telling her that it was no use—that her husband's "posse mechanism" was simply kicking in—but I thought better of it.

As the mob continued to grow, I saw Stewart shoot a panicky look toward his pregnant fiancée. A handful of policemen and security guards pressed themselves against the mob and struggled to keep order, but the crowd had a will of its own, and there was little they could do. In the tumult I took an elbow to the head, was almost shoved into Stewart's oldest daughter, and somehow ended up back next to Braunstein.

"This is awesome," she said, tears running down her cheeks. "There he is, standing by his star. I just can't believe it. I can't believe it."

Stewart and his visibly frightened family managed to make their way back to the giant stretch limo waiting by the curb. The doors slammed shut, the tires screeched, and the car sped away as a gang of desperate fans stood on their tiptoes to get one last glimpse of their idol.

That afternoon Stewart made an appearance on *Larry King Live,* after which I joined him and Penny Lancaster for a ride in their limo. "Hop in, mate," Stewart said as he walked out of the CNN studios with his arm around his fiancée. "We're headed home!" This wasn't exactly accurate. *He* was headed home. I was just riding along to ask a few questions, which was the arrangement I had negotiated with his publicist.

"That got scary back at the Walk of Fame event," Stewart said as he eased back into the plush leather seat. "I'm sort of used to it—my whole life has been a bit like that—but I was worried for my two smaller kids and, more importantly, I was worried because of Penny." Lancaster, who looked exhausted, smiled appreciatively. The paparazzi could be difficult to handle, Stewart said, but luckily his fans were always well behaved—even if some of them were a little fanatical. I asked what he thought of his more obsessive fans.

"I'm a great Glasgow Celtic fan," he said. "I wouldn't say I'm obsessed, but I get a great deal of pleasure out of collecting the programs and watching the games. It's entertainment. It's what fills our lives. And it's the same for my fans. It's what gives them happiness. So yes, I can identify with them. It's almost like an identity of sorts. People need another identity other than their own, something that they can latch on to—something that takes away the tedium."

When I asked Stewart if he knew Marcy Braunstein, he nodded vigorously. "Of course I know her—she's at every show!" he said proudly. "And she has been there, I would imagine, since the late seventies." Stewart seemed completely unfazed by Braunstein's devotion. When I mentioned that she had a Rod Room in her house, he simply nodded. I added that the room even had a shirt he had once worn.

"Oh, more than likely," he replied nonchalantly.

"And a glass of water that you once drank from."

"Yes, yes, yes. It's terribly flattering—it really is—even if it is bordering on obsession—which I have no complaints about." He smiled. "It is wonderful! And maybe if it hadn't been for Marcy, my name would not have been down on the sidewalk!"

A few minutes later the limousine rolled to a halt at a seemingly random intersection in the middle of Beverly Hills. "Well, this is the end of the line for you, mate," Stewart said, again flashing his thousand-watt smile.

"Good-bye," I mumbled, as the limo door slammed shut. The car pulled away, and I found myself alone by the side of the road.

Braunstein was overjoyed when I telephoned her that evening and told her about my conversation with Stewart. "He really knows who I am!" she said giddily. "Oh, you must send me a copy of your notes—or better yet, a tape of the interview." I assured her that I would, but as I did, I felt a pang of uneasiness: I was now playing the role of the enabler by giving her one more Rod Stewart fix. I also wondered how long it would be before Marcy was craving yet another encounter with Rod Stewart. Now that she had actually helped introduce Stewart onstage at the Walk of Fame ceremony, would she continue to be satisfied with chance encounters at crowded concerts, when he might recognize her for a fleeting moment? Or would she need a bigger fix, from visiting his house or riding with him in his limo? Braunstein, like all the other Rod Stewart fans I met, insisted that she was not and never would be a stalker. Yet many of them seemed to walk a very fine line between fandom and stalking, and I wondered if and when some of them had crossed it.

The distinction between the two is not exactly clear-cut. "Fan," which first came into popular usage during the 1880s, as a word to describe ardent baseball enthusiasts, derives from the Latin *fanaticus,* meaning "frenzied, frantic, or inspired by a deity." In the context of the entertainment business, stalkers are considered to be overzealous fans who follow, spy on, or harass celebrities. In California, at least, a stalker is legally defined as "any person who willfully, maliciously, and repeatedly . . . harasses another person and who makes a credible threat with the intent to place that person in reasonable fear for his or her safety." Thus stalkers and fans may be distinguishable not by their level of zealotry but by their respect for the privacy and well-being of the people they admire.

Some experts surmise that once an ardent fan meets his or her idol, the chances of stalking increase. Kerry Ferris, who studied encounters between Trekkies and their idols, concluded, "Once a fan acquires the ability to stage a meeting with a celebrity, the balance of power in the fan-celebrity encounter undergoes a fundamental shift. The security afforded to the celebrity by the scripts and structures of the pre-staged encounters is gone, and the element of chance is removed. As the fan gains power, the celebrity loses protection, and the specter of stalking arises."

"Skid Row" is a part of downtown Los Angeles that is so dilapidated, so overrun with squatters, and so generally devoid of civilization that if Kurt Russell wanted to make a sequel to his post-apocalyptic thriller, *Escape from L.A.,* he would be hard-pressed to find a more authentic-looking set. This is the neighborhood where the city's Threat Management Unit—informally known as "the Celebrity Anti-Stalking Unit"—is located.

A special unit of the LAPD, the TMU is run by a detective in his midforties named Jeff Dunn. The morning I visited Dunn, he was dressed with textbook neatness in slacks, a freshly pressed shirt, and a sturdy leather belt from which hung his 9 millimeter pistol, his standard-issue Smith & Wesson handcuffs, and an extra clip containing fifteen bullets. Roughly five foot eight, with a trim athletic build and reddish-blond hair, Dunn bore a vague resemblance to the former vice president Dan Quayle.

It was barely 7:00 A.M. when I met him in the lobby of his office building, and already he seemed overwhelmed by the day's work ahead. "My team works on two hundred and fifty cases a year," he said, "which may not seem like a lot compared with other units, but over here you can get bogged down quickly by the attorneys, and the chiefs, and the mayor, and all the boot-licking lackeys who are associated with high-profile people. And we're not just talking about Tom Cruise. We get cases all the time from people I've never heard of—TV stars, movie stars, rock groups, you name it—and somewhere out there, there's a fan base."

We rode the elevator up several floors and walked through a labyrinth of hulking black file cabinets, all padlocked and dusty. The whole floor smelled of burnt coffee. The floors were covered with cheap, stringy carpeting, and the walls were decorated with dog-eared posters, including one for Clint Eastwood's movie *Sudden Impact,* which boasted, "Dirty Harry is at it again."

"It's not much to look at," Dunn said as he led me back to a small conference room. "But if we need to meet with the high-profile types or the studio heads, we can do it at their place." We sat at a table in the center of the room. Dunn took out a pad and pencil and commenced a quick tutorial on the four basic types of stalkers. The most common are "simple obsessional" stalkers. These are usually neighbors, coworkers, customers, or former lovers whose prior relationship with their victims somehow turned sour. The second types are the "erotomanic stalkers" who suffer from a disorder actually listed in the *Diagnostic and Statistical Manual IV.* They have delusions that a public figure is in love with them. The third types are "love obsessional" stalkers. These are typically obsessed fans who think they might become friends with their idol, if only they could meet—and so they launch elaborate campaigns to make themselves known to the celebrity. The fourth type is the "imaginary stalker," who crops up during "false victimization syndrome," when a celebrity invents a stalker story in order to get attention. "We see that from time to time," Dunn said with a sigh. "I guess you're no one in Hollywood unless you've been stalked."

When I described my encounters with the Rod Stewart fans in detail, Dunn said that a few of them exhibited some love obsessional traits, but so far none appeared to be stalkers, because their campaign for Stewart's attention hadn't risen to the level of outright harassment. "Some of these fans clearly have impulse issues," he said. "The fact that they think they can just go to Rod Stewart's home or hotel room and maybe hang out with him is somewhat concerning." If he were doing a "threat assessment" on one of these fans, Dunn said, he would begin by looking at the "stabilizing factors"—job, spouse, family, friends— that he or she had. These factors often play a crucial role, he said—especially when they disappear: "If one of these fans lost a spouse and then felt ignored by Rod at an event, I might start to worry."

The most important issue, Dunn said, is how a celebrity feels about a given fan or would-be stalker. When I explained that Stewart didn't seem the least bit concerned about any of his fans, Dunn shrugged. "There are some things that are concerning here," he said, "but if Rod Stewart doesn't seem to mind these people doing what they do, what business is it of mine?" As he saw it, this was a good example of how tricky stalking cases could be: On the one hand, Stewart wanted to be seen as a down-to-earth, approachable person who was willing to meet his fans and sign autographs. On the other hand, he had to be wary of obsessive fans who might be looking for an excuse to show up at his house and begin harassing him.

"Everyone wants to brush with something important and

meaningful that they can attach themselves to," Dunn said. "Mark David Chapman, who killed John Lennon, said that he wanted his name forever associated with Lennon. Prior to killing him, he was a fan, and he went up to him and asked him for an autograph. The question is always 'How far is any one person willing to go?'"

There is no consensus on what turns some fans into stalkers. Some evidence suggests that childhood traumas may be to blame. Kris Mohandie has made a name for himself by overseeing and publishing the largest study of stalkers ever done, drawing on 1,005 cases, of which 271 involved public figures. Mohandie found that a significant number of stalkers had "attachment issues" dating back to childhood, when a parent either had died or hadn't given them enough love or support. "That explains some stalking behavior," Mohandie told me. "But in general, people may feel empty or powerless—for any number of reasons—and so they want to identify with some idealized person who has all the traits they covet. For them, this may be a way of lifting themselves out of the abyss. This is a way of finding relief. In that regard, I've often said that stalking is really an addiction of sorts. Often stalkers are trying to escape an unpleasant mood state. The act of stalking actually seems to fix or numb feelings of abandonment, rejection, helplessness, hopelessness, or rage. But the effect is temporary, and they soon find themselves wanting to stalk again, even though that behavior may have very adverse consequences."

Mohandie and other experts also say that there is no reliable way to identify potential stalkers. John C. Lane Jr., a retired LAPD lieutenant and the man who developed the department's Threat Management Unit, is now a partner at a consulting firm in Los Angeles called the Omega Threat Management Group. Lane keeps an eye out for rabid fans who are also social recluses. Many of his clients are local or national newscasters. According to Lane, these newscasters feel more familiar than the girl next door to many stalkers. "There is no one type of person that becomes a stalker," he says, "but often you've got these reclusive individuals who aren't married, and they're living with relatives or at a board-and-care home. And what are they doing? They're watching television constantly and developing a relationship with these newscasters whom they see two and three times a day. Many of them have never had a love interest or relationship in their real life, so they end up just taking that leap and developing these imaginary relationships."

The recluses Lane described struck me as extreme examples of the lonely Americans who read *Us Weekly* or watch *Friends* in order to fill a void in their personal lives. One could argue that the recluses are just a bit further along the same spectrum. After all, as research psychologists are quick to point out, most of us form para-social relationships with Brad Pitt and other celebrities we see on TV and in the movies. What's more, few of us would have qualms about buying a copy of Bill Gordon's *The Ultimate Hollywood Guide* and using it to drive by or perhaps even stake out Pitt's home for a few minutes. So how surprising is it that some people are willing to go a step further and hop the fence into Brad Pitt's backyard?

"I guess I am feeling a bit down," Marcy Braunstein told me when we met one last time in the lobby of the Roosevelt Hotel. It was just a day after the Walk of Fame ceremony, but all her giddiness was gone, and in its place was an almost melancholy calm. She eventually confided that she was feeling very out of place here in Hollywood. "When I looked at some of the pictures of the ceremony that our friends took," she said, "you see Rod is all dazzling and I am just plain Jane. I realize I don't belong here. I'm never going to have the money or the fame or the stature that Rod has. There isn't a chance that I will ever be part of his inner circle. Of course, I've felt this way before, but I felt it more than usual yesterday."

According to Linda Kay, the former president of the National Association of Fan Clubs, devoted fans are often looking for a way to connect with their idols. "You don't hear many fan-club presidents admit this out loud," she said, "but I think some of them hope that their position will help them meet and even befriend their celebrities. When you're a fan-club president, you really do feel this sense of connection. You are the nexus for all this information and fan activity, and sometimes you feel like you are a part of the celebrity's world." In Kay's experience, most fan-club presidents know how and when to draw the line between themselves and the celebrities they admire. Those who don't set themselves up for a "major letdown."

"I would never want to wish away the affection I have for Rod," Braunstein told me at the Roosevelt Hotel. "I enjoy the emotion—and in order to have the highs you have to have the lows." She fell silent for a moment, as if lost in thought, and when she began speaking again, her voice was barely audible. "When I saw Rod dancing around on the star, that did make me cry," she said. "I was happy for him. I've certainly said enough times that everyone has to have their baby."

I asked her why she'd never had children.

"Some people think that it's the interracial thing, because I am white and Dave is black, but it has nothing to do with that," she replied. "I just had such a terrible childhood that I never wanted to have children. I just never viewed childhood as being very positive. I came from a family that was dysfunctional—a family where, as a child, I had to build up some mental defenses. My mother did not encourage us to express emotion, and boy, this Rod stuff is emotion. I guess I didn't get a whole lot of love or acknowledgment as a kid, and that's something I seek when I go to a Rod concert."

Later I spoke with Braunstein's older brother, Michael, who helped me better understand her need for recognition. "My mother was a fanatical disciplinarian, and she was very hard to get to know," he told me over the phone. "She was never one to give out accolades or praise to the children. You could never make this woman happy. No matter how hard you worked, it wasn't hard enough. And no matter how good it was, it was never good enough. I guess that's why all of us siblings have this need to be acknowledged. That is why, more than anything else,

I like to hear my boss say, 'Yeah, Michael, you did a nice job.'"

Marcy Braunstein's dissatisfaction with the Walk of Fame ceremony was short-lived. Not long after our final meeting at the Roosevelt Hotel, she set out for Stewart's house again. Her plan was to ask Stewart to sign a few pieces of memorabilia for her Rod Room. When she arrived at the inner gates to his mansion she announced her name into an intercom, and slowly—almost magically—the gates opened. Braunstein proceeded cautiously, clutching the steering wheel with one hand and snapping photos with the other. At the top of the driveway a personal assistant emerged from the house and explained that Stewart was in the shower but that he would gladly sign the memorabilia and mail it back to her.

"So it all worked out," she told me later. "And I felt much better."

Conclusion: Some Reflections from Hollywood's Premier Retirement Home

In Woodland Hills, California, is a sprawling retirement community known simply as The Fund. The community, which is run by the Motion Picture and Television Fund, opens its doors to all actors, directors, costume designers, makeup artists, gaffers, soundmen, and other professionals from the industry who have grown too old or infirm to take care of themselves. This cloistered enclave in the foothills of the Santa Monica Mountains is the last stop for many of the men and women who once ran Hollywood.

On my visit to The Fund, I parked alongside one hospital wing, the George Burns Intensive Care Unit. I then headed down a small path, which took me past Harry's Haven—a gated complex for Alzheimer's patients, funded by Kirk Douglas and named after his father—and into a park with spreading lawns and dozens of swaying sycamore trees. Dotting this landscape were quaint cottages in which some of the more mobile residents lived. The campus had all the trappings of a tidy, fully functioning small town in the Midwest, including a library, a grand old cinema with weekly screenings, and a one-room chapel with five rows of benches and a few stained-glass windows.

I walked into a modern building with a large cafeteria and soon came upon an elderly couple who invited me to join them for lunch. The woman, a former actress named Liz Fraser, was in her eighties, though there was still a certain youthful vitality in her face that revealed the ingénue she'd played in Hollywood during the 1940s. The man—who wore Velcro sneakers, two hearing aids, and a Kangol hat—introduced himself as Gerry O'Loughlin, a lifelong character actor. "I'm still working," he told me. "And I'm eighty-three . . . No, I'm eighty-six . . . No, I'm eighty-two." We all kept silent for a moment. "Actually, I'm eighty-three. Thank God I got that straight."

O'Loughlin explained that despite his advancing years, he had just auditioned for a spin-off of *Star Trek*. He didn't generally like such programs—he said the thought of all that "pseudo-Shakespearean dialogue" made him want to vomit. Nonetheless, he had agreed to audition for the part because he wanted to impress his new manager, who had only recently agreed to represent him. "I played a Vulcan or some kind of big shot on another planet," O'Loughlin said. "And he makes this speech that just about killed me. It goes"—he cleared his throat—"Student of Seron . . . um, oh shit, okay . . . Student of Seron, who said logic is the cement of our civilization with which we ascend from chaos using reason as our guide." He sighed heavily. "Now, that speech needed to be rattled off, and I couldn't do it. I had ample time to learn it, but I just couldn't."

Moments later, Robert Guillaume, who starred in the TV show *Benson,* walked past us and headed over to a seat at the far end of the dining hall. "That's Robert," Fraser said casually when he was out of earshot. "He was a fine actor."

"I know," I replied. "I recognized him immediately."

Fraser and O'Loughlin exchanged a quick glance of frustration, as if this was not the first time they had been eclipsed by Guillaume.

A server took our lunch orders, and while we waited for the food to arrive, Fraser told me more about her career, which had included major roles in *The Man Who Came to Dinner* (1942), *All My Sons* (1948), *Death of a Salesman* (1951), *Young at Heart* (1954), *Tunnel of Love* (1958), *A Patch of Blue* (1965), and many others.

"You should have seen her back then," O'Loughlin said admiringly. "Go have a look—her picture is on the Wall."

"What wall?" I asked.

"*The* Wall," Fraser said. She pointed to the far side of the dining hall, where her photograph hung with those of O'Loughlin and all the other residents. Many of the photos were black-and-white headshots from the 1940s and 1950s, when the residents were at the height of their careers. They were the sort of glamour shots that stars today still sign and send out to fans. "I don't spend too much time looking at the Wall," one resident told me later. "It gets frightening when you see yourself back then." Fraser's photo showed a cute buxom blonde who might have passed for a young Dolly Parton. I complimented her on it and asked when it had been taken.

"In 1864," O'Loughlin said with a laugh. "Just after the Battle of Bull Run."

"It was taken in the 1950s," Fraser said. "And you should look at it all you want, because I don't pose for photographs anymore."

Later on she told me why. "I'm ugly," she said. "Inside, I still think I'm Lana Turner, but I look at pictures of myself today and I think, *You're fat, your face is much too big, and I hate your hair.* I'm attractive for eighty-four, but I sure as shit ain't attractive."

This confession was followed by a long silence.

"Now's your chance to tell me I'm not right," she said with a sad smile.

"You're not right," I stammered.

"The funny thing is," she said, "when I was young, I had no idea that I was pretty. Then I got to a certain age and I realized: *You had it—you had it all.*"

I was often reminded in Woodland Hills of the A. E. Housman poem "To an Athlete Dying Young," in which the narrator suggests that his friend, an accomplished runner, was lucky to die young, while he was still at the top of his game. Housman writes: "Now you will not swell the rout / Of lads that wore their honours out, / Runners whom renown outran / And the name died before the man."

The sad truth of the matter is that few elderly celebrities get as much attention as their younger counterparts, or ever win Academy Awards. Jessica Tandy, who at the age of eighty won an Oscar for best actress in 1989, for *Driving Miss Daisy,* is an exception. According to Douglas Kenrick, of Arizona State University, who has studied the ages of Hollywood entertainers, the median age of Oscar-winning actors between 1950 and 2004 was forty-two for men and thirty-three and a half for women. Even when elderly actors are nominated, they rarely receive much press. Janice Min, the editor of *Us Weekly,* says, "You might have a really fine actress like Judi Dench who gets nominated for an Oscar, but those aren't the sort of people who draw the buzz and the heat." As far as the media is concerned, most award shows have simply become opportunities to gush over celebrities—especially young celebrities. *Us Weekly*'s coverage of the 2005 MTV Video Music Awards, for example, focused on the fact that Nicky Hilton (then twenty-one) had dyed her hair blond, that Jessica Simpson (twenty-five) wore a scandalous version of a French maid's outfit, and that Kirsten Dunst (twenty-three) was getting intimate with Orlando Bloom (twenty-eight). "These award shows are really just becoming celebrations of fame and youth," Min concludes.

The preeminent celebration of this kind, of course, is the official pre-show for the Academy Awards, during which all the nominees arrive by limo. Nielsen Media Research found that approximately 27.7 million Americans watched this half-hour program in 2005—more than watched the seventh game of the 2005 NBA finals, the 2005 Miss America Pageant, and Ken Burns's series on jazz combined. In fact, the show was so popular that ABC decided to lengthen it to an hour in 2006. According to Dennis Doty, who has been producing the show since its inception, in 1999, this popularity makes perfect sense: "You look at all the programming that dwells on fame and show business—like *Entertainment Tonight, Access Hollywood, The In-*

sider—and this is the culmination of that. Basically, this is the moment when our idealized notion of glamour comes to fruition." Interestingly, *nothing* really happens on the pre-show: we simply watch celebrities parading around. And in a way this seems to be how we like them best—not when they're acting, or singing, or making speeches but when they're walking down the red carpet, looking young and beautiful, and letting us imagine just how marvelous all this must be.

Ultimately, our obsession with celebrities isn't about them; it's about *us* and *our* needs. Many of us look at these people—who have glamour, beauty, wealth, and youth—and familiarize ourselves with them until they begin to feel like real people in our lives. We discuss them at work, in the park, and over dinner. We develop feelings for them. We love them, or hate them, or pity them, or profess not to care but secretly do. In one way or another we use them. And when they grow old and lose the traits that once made them noteworthy—when they become frail, aged mortals like the residents of The Fund—we conveniently forget them, because they no longer serve our needs.

One afternoon in Woodland Hills, I bumped into Hal Riddle—an eighty-five-year-old former character actor with a bushy mustache and gentle, baggy eyes. He was wearing a crisp brown Members Only jacket that looked as if it had just been taken out of a hermetically sealed capsule. "Let's go back to my room," Riddle said. "We can talk there for a while." Riddle, who got around via an electric scooter, motioned for me to follow him and then sped down a long hallway. Riddle's room was a cozy place furnished with an antique Chippendale chair, a roll-top desk, a bookshelf crammed with books on acting, and a window overlooking a tomato farm and the distant Santa Monica Mountains.

"I grew up in Calhoun, Kentucky," Riddle said as he settled into a chair. "And I'll tell you what: when you grow up there, Hollywood seems like a wonderful, far-off, never-never land—a place of beauty and riches and everything else." He recalled when his father had taken him to see his very first movie, a saga about the life of Jesse James. His father's intention was to dissuade him from ever contemplating a life of crime, but what the boy took away from this outing was that he wanted to become a movie star. "I remember that the audience was applauding these actors, and in my heart I wanted to be up there on that screen too."

When he was a young man, Riddle moved to New York City and found work as an actor in the theater. His first Broadway appearance was a supporting role in *Mister Roberts;* his performance often earned a round of applause when he exited the stage. The first time this happened, he was overwhelmed: "I almost felt like a child who gets up and sings his ABCs for the first time and the teacher pats him on the head and says, 'Very good—you learned them all.'" Eventually he moved to Hollywood, where he landed minor parts in a number of movies, including several with Elvis Presley. He remembers being desperate to have Elvis's fame. "Elvis got everything he prayed for and I didn't," he said with a smile. Then he added quietly, almost to himself, "Then again, look how things turned out for Elvis."

Riddle strove throughout his career to become a movie star, but the only parts he got were small supporting roles. He appeared on television in *Charlie's Angels, Little House on the Prairie,* and *The Mary Tyler Moore Show,* but nothing ever turned him into a household name. Still, he worked hard, and never found time for a wife and family along the way. According to Riddle, his one true love was a girl from Fulton, Kentucky, named Lillian. They attended high school together in the late 1930s, and Riddle was smitten. Unfortunately, his feelings were unrequited. "I've often wondered, if I had been able to win over Lillian, whether my love for her would have transcended my desire for fame," he told me. "You know, most actors say that they need to express themselves, but fame is really the spur. We want to be accepted. We are really begging people, 'Accept me!' Let's face it—it's all about wanting to be loved."

In his older years Riddle clung to the hope that fame was

still within his grasp. He looked for encouragement from actors who'd made it late in life. In the late 1980s he took heart when Claire Peller gained fame as the crotchety old woman in the Wendy's "Where's the beef?" commercials.

"You see," he said finally, "fame is really an addiction. And when it takes you as a child, and when you build on it your whole life, even if you look around and all you see is ruins, you can't leave the ruins. Alcoholics Anonymous says that when you get sober, you're still a 'sober alcoholic.' You may no longer drink, but the alcoholic personality is still there, and it will be there until you die. You just aren't feeding it with anything. It's the same thing with me. I'm out of the business, but I'll never be completely out of the business, because inside I still dream about it —I just don't feed it."

During my time at The Fund I talked with other residents who hoped they might still achieve the fame that had so far eluded them. But some, like Audrey Totter, insisted that they were thoroughly finished. In the 1940s Totter was one of Hollywood's most glamorous starlets. She played alongside Lana Turner in *The Postman Always Rings Twice,* and starred with Robert Montgomery in *Lady in the Lake.* When she quit acting, in her late twenties, she had appeared in more than three dozen movies.

I met Totter, a slight woman with curly white hair and watery blue eyes, one evening after dinner. She was sitting by herself on a couch in the lobby with a cane across her lap and an emergency-alert button hanging from her neck like a plastic medallion. When I introduced myself, she extended a long, slender hand distinguished by a handsome turquoise ring. We chatted for a while, and I asked her what it was like being a starlet back in the 1940s. She told me about a trip to New York City when her clothes were literally torn off. "I was in front of the hotel— at the Plaza, in fact—and all these people rushed to get autographs, and they pulled off my clothes, and a policeman took off his coat and put it around me and took me back into the hotel. They were tearing at my dress for souvenirs."

Totter was quick to add that her fame ended when she quit acting. "I met a doctor whom I fell madly in love with at first sight, and when he asked me to marry him, of course I said yes, and I gave up my career. We were married for forty-two years, which I think is a record out here in Hollywood."

"Did you have any regrets about what you gave up?" I asked.

"Not at all. I've had a wonderful marriage, children, and grandchildren, and how many people out here can say that?"

The following day, when I caught up again with Hal Riddle, I told him I'd met Totter. "Yeah, Audrey just up and walked away," he said. He speculated that she'd done so because she had the "nesting instinct," which most men don't have. He'd always thought he would have time for a wife and family once he became famous. "I suppose part of me wanted to drop the pursuit of fame," he added. "But something down deep wouldn't let me. Fame is like a mistress in that way. You try to turn away, but the mistress always says, 'Come back and try one more time.' She always offers you delights. And you just swear you're never going to see her again, because you've got a wife or a family—or you want one—but the lure of the mistress is always there."

Toward the end of our conversation I asked Riddle about the future. "Do you still think it could happen for you?" I asked. "Could you still become famous?"

"Oh, boy," he said with a chortle. "My first question would be 'Does the part have any lines?' Because I don't want to learn lines anymore, or worry about them in the back of my mind. I've never told anyone this, but I think if there could be a part where I'm totally mute—I mean I don't have to say anything for the role, I just have to express everything that comes across my whole being—then I think I could do it. Of course, I don't walk as well as I used to, but you know, we can cover that up. My character could be an old man or an invalid. Yes, I think I could do it. In fact, I think I'd win an Academy Award."

The odd thing about Riddle's conviction that he was "addicted to fame" is that by his own admission, he was never famous.

What he couldn't tear himself away from was not fame, per se, but the *pursuit* of fame. What's more, this may have prevented him from starting a family and having a more robust personal life, but it did not greatly damage or destroy him. For this reason addiction experts like Dr. Nora Volkow, of the National Institute for Drug Abuse, would be quick to argue that Riddle's obsession was not an addiction in the purest, clinical sense of the word.

In all likelihood, there are *not* a great many people whose lives have been completely ruined by their obsession with fame. But many people seem willing to pay a considerable price — parting with their spouses, quitting their jobs, leaving their homes, humiliating themselves on reality TV, or even sharing their most intimate secrets with a TV talk-show host — in order to get the rush that comes from being in the spotlight. Indeed, in my estimation, the people in all three of the niches I have explored in this book may be paying a far greater price for their relationship with fame than they think.

For the casual observers who follow the lives of celebrities, the price may be the least obvious. After all, what's the harm in keeping tabs on Brad Pitt's life from time to time? Perhaps the best way to answer this question is to consider the events of a single day: January 7, 2005. On that day the table of contents on page A2 of the *New York Times* listed a number of serious news stories including [1] a breakthrough in AIDS research by scientists in Texas, [2] a new plan by the Bush administration to rescue the federal pension-insurance program, [3] a surprising decision by Senator Max Baucus of Montana to oppose President Bush's Social Security plan, [4] an early glimpse at Paul Volcker's investigation into the UN's scandalous oil-for-food program, and [5] the dismissal of charges against a Chinese-American woman named Katrina Leung who was accused of using a sexual relationship with an FBI agent to secure national military documents. Yet one of the most widely reported stories of the day, particularly on TV news, had nothing to do with any of these. Here is how Greta Van Susteren of Fox News broke this story: "This is a Fox News alert. Hollywood power couple Jennifer Aniston and Brad Pitt have separated after four and one half years of marriage . . ." The following day CNN's *Saturday Morning News* also reported this story. A word-count analysis of CNN transcripts for that day and the following one reveals that the network devoted more coverage to Pitt and Aniston than to the combined total of the five real news stories mentioned above.

Andrew Tyndall, author of the online *Tyndall Report*, studies the content of television news. It was Tyndall who drew attention to the fact that in 2004 the nightly news shows on the three major networks spent a total of just 26 minutes covering the bloody conflict in Darfur and 130 minutes on the Martha Stewart scandal. (In 2005 the total coverage of Darfur on these three shows dropped to just eighteen minutes.) When it comes to airing "celebrity news" instead of "hard news," Tyndall says that the morning shows and the daytime cable news shows are the real culprits. He notes that in 2004 the three network morning shows—*Good Morning America,* the *Today* show, and *The Early Show*—devoted more minutes of coverage to the Michael Jackson trial than to the 9/11 Commission report or the abuse of prisoners at Abu Ghraib or the death of the former president Ronald Reagan. In fact, *Good Morning America* and *The Early Show* gave about as much coverage to Michael Jackson and Martha Stewart combined as to the war in Iraq. According to Tyndall, during major events in the news cycle, such as the flooding of New Orleans and the capture of Saddam Hussein, these shows stick to the "hard news." But during the lulls—which encompass 90 percent of news days, in Tyndall's estimation—they are awash with celebrity news and true-crime stories. And this trend, he concludes, shows no sign of changing.

The many Americans who clamor to get near celebrities also pay a price. According to Robert Cialdini, of Arizona State University, "basking in reflected glory" presents something of a trap for those who make a practice of it. Although BIRGing provides a quick and relatively safe way for people with low self-esteem to feel better about themselves, some people can become addicted to the process and eventually feel that their own success—indeed, their sense of self-worth—depends entirely on their connections to the famous and successful. Young people may be at greatest risk. In the Rochester survey 43.4 percent of teenage girls said they wanted to become celebrity personal assistants when they grew up. They chose this option twice as often as "the president of a great university like Harvard or Yale," three times as often as "a United States Senator," and four times as often as "the chief of a major company like General Motors." What's so interesting about this statistic is that among girls who said they received bad grades—C or below—in school, the percentage who opted to become assistants rose to 67 percent. What's more, among both boys and girls who got bad grades—and also described themselves as unpopular at school—the percentage who opted to become assistants rose further to 80 percent. As these teenagers mature, of course, many of them will develop other professional goals. Yet if even a small fraction of them pursue their current aspirations, vast numbers of young people may soon be flocking to L.A. and New York in hopes of enhancing their self-esteem by working intimately with celebrities. Josef Csongei, the president of the Association of Celebrity Personal Assistants, says this is highly problematic. "I could see how teenagers, and even perhaps some adults, would see this kind of job as a way of being acknowledged, recognized, and respected," he told me. "But I don't think any job is really going to make you feel better about yourself. The only person who can make you feel better about yourself is *you*. This is internal work. And no outside person, celebrity or not, can do that for you."

Finally, when it comes to those who are seeking fame directly, there is also a price to be paid. Again, those who stand to pay most dearly are young people. Some of the most disturbing findings in the Rochester survey came from the portion in which participants were asked to describe what good fame might do them and how celebrities made them feel. Many described fame as an almost magical solution to all the problems that life might present. One eighth-grade boy wrote, "I would never have to worry about the things I have to now. My family would have money and people would respect me more. I would finally be realized." A sixth-grade boy said, "The best thing about being famous is the pride. You would probably have more self-confidence in yourself. You'd feel important." And one seventh-grade girl wrote, "Celebrities make me jealous, because they have everything. They are really pretty and perfect and smart! I want to be them. Make me them!" These statements may help explain why—when given the option to become stronger, smarter, famous, or more beautiful—boys in the survey chose fame almost as often as intelligence, and girls chose it more often.

The fascination that young people have with the notion of becoming famous does not appear to be waning. The best proof of this may be the continuing popularity of *American Idol,* which began its fifth season in January of 2006. In the history of television no reality-TV shows—and very few programs of any kind—have ever enjoyed a significant increase in ratings during a fifth season. Yet viewers for the 2006 season premiere increased by 10 percent from the previous year, reaching 35.5 million. Much of this success can be attributed to young people. The *New York Times* noted, "Among teenage girls, the show had an extraordinary forty-nine share—meaning that of every girl in the country watching television for those two hours, with about one hundred channels to choose from in most homes, half were watching Fox [which broadcasts *American Idol*]." There is good reason to believe that many of these teenagers not only hope for but expect fame at some point in their lives. According to a Washington Post/Kaiser Family Foundation/Harvard University survey conducted in 2005, 31 percent of American teenagers think they will become famous one day.

Of course, the pursuit of fame isn't necessarily dubious or unhealthy. For those young people who truly are talented—or at least have the promise of talent—going to auditions in front of judges, scouts, and agents may be a rewarding experience. It may even open the door to a successful career as an entertainer.

Yet anyone who has watched the first round of an *American Idol* competition, or stepped into the lobby at an IMTA convention, can see the painful and obvious truth that for every talented contestant there are masses of others who appear to have nothing but a desperate desire for fame and everything it promises to bestow.

Keith Campbell, of the University of Georgia, has spent years studying the psychology of narcissism and entitlement. To him the fact that so many teenagers expect to become famous is very troublesome. Starting in the mid-1990s Campbell conducted extensive research using the Narcissism Personality Inventory. His findings suggest that American teenagers have very high levels of narcissism and entitlement compared with older Americans and compared with teenagers from other parts of the world. Campbell fears that in America, because fame appears so readily available on TV and elsewhere, the atmosphere fosters narcissism and entitlement. Basically, adolescents everywhere have delusions of fame and grandeur, but in America these thoughts don't seem so far-fetched. The danger with this, insists Campbell, is that teenagers are essentially being encouraged to adopt the prima donna's mindset—in which they are constantly looking to be admired—because, after all, they believe their own fame is imminent.

Perhaps needless to say, the vast majority are in for a big disappointment. In fact, they may soon find themselves empathizing with Tyler Durden, the character in Chuck Palahniuk's novel *Fight Club,* who says, "We are the middle children of history, raised by television to believe that someday we'll be millionaires and movie stars and rock stars, but we won't. And we're just learning this fact . . . So don't fuck with us." Admittedly, it's troubling to contemplate a generation of Americans who are bitter that they never became famous. But more troubling is the alternative: namely, a generation clinging forever to the hope that any day now they will get the recognition, admiration, and fame they are due.

• • •

After my visit to Woodland Hills, I was overcome by an urge to call Eddie and Wyatt Powell, in Battle Mountain, Nevada. It had been half a year since I'd met them at the IMTA convention in Los Angeles, and I was curious to see how they were doing. Wyatt answered the phone and told me that Eddie was doing fine, even though no agents had expressed any interest in representing him. Cal Merlander had offhandedly suggested that Eddie take some private acting lessons and then get back in touch with him. This had given Eddie a glimmer of hope, and he was lobbying for his father to take him back to L.A. in a few months. "We'll probably pursue it," Wyatt said. "But I don't know where to draw the line between what he wants and reality. We were way unrealistic with the money that we invested, but on the other hand, I don't want to be cheap. I guess we'll do it because, as I've said, you've got to support your kids."

When I spoke with Eddie, he was quick to tell me that all was well at school. "When I got back to school, every single person was asking me how it went, and I just told them that the acting business takes a lot of time and I probably wouldn't be famous until we're in eighth grade, which is a long time from now. By then I will have gone out to L.A. and met with that agent again."

"How did the kids react to that?" I asked.

"Well," he said, "they think it still might happen a year from now, so they want to stay on my good side. In fact, the day I came back, about twenty kids asked me for my autograph. I guess they wanted to be able to say 'I knew this guy before he was famous.'"

Note on Name Changes

In order to protect the identity of some of the people in this book, I have changed their names and hometowns. This includes all the children and teenagers in chapters 1 through 3 and their parents and grandparents; Jill Marlin in chapter 2; Cal Merlander, the agent, and his company, Glamour Talent, in chapter 2, chapter 3, and the conclusion; Annie Brentwell and her parents in chapter 4; and Marcel Winter, the stylist, in chapter 6.

Appendix: The Rochester Survey

I. Overview

The Rochester survey was written by Jake Halpern and Professor Carol M. Liebler, a professor at Syracuse University. Most of its thirty-two questions related to fame and pop culture. Copies of the survey were distributed to 653 students at three schools in and around Rochester, New York. The students were fifth-, sixth-, seventh-, and eighth-graders. Meredith Hight, a graduate student at Syracuse's Newhouse School of Public Communications, entered the data into an SPSS database. Summary responses were tabulated by Professor Elaine Allen, of Babson College. Professor Allen segmented the results by demographic information and by key variables including loneliness and amount of television viewing, among others. Analyses were examined using chi-squared statistics, with results having a p-value less than 0.05 determined to be statistically significant. (Statistical significance implies a relationship between the categories being compared.) These results were then reviewed and confirmed by Professor Richard McGowan, of Boston College. The details and methodology of this study are explained below.

II. Why Rochester, New York?

In 2004 Josh Herman, who works for a company called Acxiom, ranked those cities whose consumer demographics are most closely reflective of the United States as a whole for his "Mirror on America" study. To do this he used a system called Personicx, which analyzes such demographic information as age, marital status, home ownership, number of children, estimated income, net worth, and "urbanicity" (whether a subject lives in the city, the suburbs, or the countryside).

Personicx is used primarily by marketers who want to better understand the "consumer landscape" of a given city. Admittedly, the Acxiom study is not a perfectly ideal tool for measuring the demographics of American cities—in the way the U.S. Census Bureau does, for example—because it omits such factors as race, national origin, and religion.

Nonetheless, it provides a strong indication of which cities are most quintessentially American, and Herman compiled a list of the top 150. Rochester, New York, ranks second on his list.

III. The Schools Surveyed

One school in the city of Rochester and two in the suburbs participated in this study. In all three of these schools a "passive consent" protocol was used. In other words, no permission slips were required. All students automatically participated in the survey unless their parents actively requested that they not do so. According to school officials, no parents objected.

1. *Monroe High School* (Rochester School District): This school has 1,192 students. The survey was given to eighth-graders during class time. Monroe has a high percentage of poor and minority students, and the total nonwhite population is 88.1 percent. The poverty rate at the school—defined by the number of students who are eligible for a free or a reduced-price lunch—is 89.1 percent.

2. *Twelve Corners Middle School* (Brighton School District): This school has 865 students. The survey was given to students in the sixth, seventh, and eighth grades during health and "home and career" classes. Twelve Corners students are 75.8 percent Caucasian/White, 10.4 percent Asian, 6.8 percent Black/African American, and 3.1 percent Hispanic/Latino.

3. *Willink Middle School* (Webster School District): This school has 1,100 students. The survey was given to students in grades six through eight in classes and during study halls. Willink's students are 93.3 percent Caucasian/White, 6.6 percent Hispanic/Latino, 3.1 percent Black/African American, and 1.8 percent Asian.

IV. Demographic Information on the Participants

Of the 653 students who participated in the study, 312 were male, 310 were female, and 31 did not indicate their gender. Two students were in the fifth grade, 76 in the sixth grade, 165 in the seventh grade, and 377 in the eighth grade; 33 subjects did not indicate their grade. They included 329 who were white/Caucasian, 95 mixed-race, 62 black/African American, 58 Hispanic/Latino, and 14 Native American; 95 students did not indicate their race.

V. Explanation of All Findings Quoted in This Book

1. Going to Fame School

p. 12 "The teenagers who regularly watch certain celebrity-focused TV shows—*Entertainment Tonight, Access Hollywood,* and *The Insider*—are more likely than others to believe that they themselves will be famous someday."

Methodology: This was determined in relatively simple fashion. Question #7 asked students whether they put their chances of becoming famous above or below 50 percent. Question #9 asked how often they watched shows like *Entertainment Tonight, Access Hollywood,* and *The Insider.* The options were never, once a month, once a week, or every day. Of those who never watched these shows, only 34 percent said they had at least a 50 percent chance of becoming famous. Of those who watched once a month, 48 percent said so. Of those who watched once a week, again 48 percent said so. And of those who watched every day, 65 percent said so.

p. 12 "The same appears to be true for teenagers who read magazines like *Us Weekly, Star, People, Teen People, YM,* and *J-14.*"

Methodology: Question #10 on the survey asked, "On average, how often do you read magazines like *Us Weekly, Star, People, Teen People, YM,* or *J-14*?" Of those who never read these magazines, 43.4 percent said they had at least a 50 percent chance of becoming famous. Of those who read once a month, 38.4 percent said so. Of those who read them once a week, 50 percent said so. And of those who read them every day, 57.6 percent said so.

p. 12 "Among those teens who watched one hour or less of TV a day, only 15 percent of the boys and 17 percent of the girls chose fame.

But among those who watched five hours or more a day—and many did—29 percent of the boys and 37 percent of the girls chose fame."

Methodology: This is a cross study of results from questions #1 and #3.

p. 13 "A number of teens commented that such stories made them feel they could and would become famous."

Methodology: This is a sampling of the written responses to question #11.

p. 22 "Teenagers in the Rochester survey were asked to choose the most likely explanation for why certain celebrities were so successful. Their options included luck, innate talent, hard work, and even the possibility that the entertainment industry simply decided to turn certain people into stars. More teenagers chose 'hard work' than all the other options combined."

Methodology: These results come from question #8, on which 9.7 percent chose luck, 42.3 percent chose hard work, 13.5 percent chose innate talent, and 7.7 chose arbitrariness in the entertainment industry. Option (e) was I'm not sure (19.4 percent). I did not include option (e) when I said "all of the other options combined."

3. A Home for the Famous and the Almost Famous

p. 71 "Teens who described themselves as often or always depressed were more likely than others to believe that becoming a celebrity would make them happier."

Methodology: Question #27 asked, "Do you ever feel depressed, and if so, how often?" The options were rarely or never, sometimes, pretty often, and almost always. Question #2 asked, "Do you think that becoming a celebrity—like a movie star or a rock star—would make you happier?" The options were yes, no, I am not sure. Of those who described themselves as rarely or never and sometimes depressed, 25 percent thought fame would make them happier. Of those who described themselves as often or always depressed, 35 percent thought fame would make them happier.

p. 71 "Those who described themselves as feeling lonely were also more likely to believe that fame would have a positive impact on their lives—though the results were slightly different between boys and girls: lonely boys were more likely to say that fame would simply make them happy, whereas lonely girls were more likely to say it would make them better liked by kids at school."

Methodology: Question #28 asked, "Do you ever feel lonely, and if so, how often?" The options were rarely or never, sometimes, pretty often, and almost always. We categorized the first two choices as "not lonely" and the last two as "lonely." Question #2 asked, "Do you think that becoming a celebrity—like a movie star or a rock star—would make you happier?" Among not lonely boys, 27 percent answered "yes," whereas 40 percent of lonely boys answered "yes." (The results were less striking among girls: 22 percent of not lonely girls answered "yes," and 28 percent of lonely girls answered "yes.") Question #16 asked, "If you became a celebrity, would kids at school like you more?" The options were probably not, maybe, definitely, and not sure. Among not lonely girls 24 percent answered "maybe" or "definitely," whereas 44 percent of lonely girls did so. (On this question the results among boys were far less striking.)

p. 71 "African American kids were more eager for fame than their peers."

Methodology: These statistics were derived by crossing the data from questions 3, 17, and 30.

p. 72 "Those who watch at least five hours of television a day are significantly more likely than those who watch just an hour or less to agree with the statement 'Becoming a celebrity [will] make you happier.'"

Methodology: Question #1 asked the respondents how many hours of television they watched per day. Of those who watched one hour or less, only 24 percent answered "yes" to Question #2 ("Do you think that becoming a celebrity—like a movie star or a rock star—would make you happier?") Of those who watched five hours or more, 37 percent answered "yes."

p. 72 "They are also twice as likely as those who watch an hour or less to believe that their families will love them more if they become celebrities."

Methodology: Question #17 asked, "If you became a celebrity, would your family love you more?" The options were probably not, maybe, definitely, and not sure. Among those teens who watched one hour or less of television per day, 11 percent said "definitely." Among those who watched five hours or more per day, 23 percent said "definitely."

5. The Desire to Belong: Why Everyone Wants to Have Dinner with Paris Hilton and 50 Cent

p. 116 "Boys who described themselves as lonely were almost twice as likely as others to endorse the statement 'My favorite celebrity just helps me feel good and forget about all of my troubles.' Girls who described themselves as lonely were almost three times as likely as others to endorse that statement."

Methodology: First we divided students into two groups: lonely and not lonely (see second note for chapter 3 on page 203). Question #22 asked, "Which of the following reasons BEST explains why you keep track of your favorite celebrity?" The options were: "(a) I just like watching this celebrity perform"; "(b) I like to imagine myself hanging out with my favorite celebrity"; "(c) My favorite celebrity just helps me feel good and forget about all of my troubles"; and "(d) I don't have a favorite celebrity." We found that 21 percent of lonely boys, compared with just 11 percent of not lonely boys, chose option (c); and 50 percent of lonely girls, compared with just 17 percent of not lonely girls, chose option (c). Both boys and girls categorized as not lonely were likelier to say either that they didn't have a favorite celebrity or that they simply liked watching their favorite celebrity perform.

p. 116 "Another survey question asked teens whom they would most like to meet for dinner: Jesus Christ, Albert Einstein, Shaquille O'Neal, Jennifer Lopez, 50 Cent, Paris Hilton, or President Bush. Among boys who said they were not lonely, the clear winner was Jesus Christ; but among those who described themselves as lonely, Jesus finished last and 50 Cent was the clear winner."

Methodology: Of those boys who described themselves as not lonely, 12 percent chose 50 Cent and 27 percent chose Jesus. Of those who described themselves as lonely, just 7 percent chose Jesus and 21 percent chose 50 Cent.

p. 117 "Similarly, girls who felt appreciated by their parents, friends, and teachers tended to choose dinner with Jesus, whereas those who felt underappreciated were likely to choose Paris Hilton."

Methodology: Question #12 asked, "How appreciated do you feel by your parents, friends, and teachers?" The options were "(a) I feel VERY appreciated"; "(b) I am basically appreciated enough"; "(c) In truth, I am NOT appreciated enough"; and "(d) It seems like hardly anyone realizes my gifts or appreciates me." Those teens who chose (a) or (b) went into the "appreciated" category, and those who chose (c) or (d) went into the "underappreciated" category. We then determined that 36 percent of appreciated girls opted for dinner with Jesus Christ, 15 percent for dinner with 50 Cent, and 15 percent for dinner with Jennifer Lopez. Meanwhile, 35 percent of underappreciated girls opted for dinner with Paris Hilton, 29 percent for dinner with 50 Cent, and 16 percent for dinner with Jesus Christ.

Conclusion

p. 195 "Among girls who said they received bad grades—C or below—in school, the percentage who opted to become assistants rose to 67 percent."

Methodology: This statistic was derived by crossing the data from questions #3 and #24.

p. 195 "Among both boys and girls who got bad grades—and also described themselves as unpopular at school—the percentage who opted to become assistants rose further to 80 percent."

Methodology: This statistic was derived by crossing the data from questions #3, #24, and #14. Question #14 asked, "At your school, how popular do you feel?" The options were: "(a) among the least popular"; "(b) below average"; "(c) average"; "(d) above average"; "(e) among the most popular"; and "(f) I don't care to say." We categorized those who picked (a) and (b) as "unpopular."

p. 196 ". . . when given the option to become stronger, smarter, famous, or more beautiful—boys in the survey chose fame almost as often as intelligence, and girls chose it more often."

Methodology: Among the boys, 23 percent chose intelligence and 19 percent chose fame. Among the girls, 20 percent chose intelligence and 24 percent chose fame.

VI. The Survey

From Jake Halpern, writer:

Survey on Beliefs and Attitudes Toward Fame

This is a <u>confidential</u> survey. No one will ever know how you responded. Please do not mark your name or any other identifiable information on this survey.

1. On average, how much television do you watch a day? *Please circle just one.*
   a) 1 hour or less
   b) 1–2 hours
   c) 3–4 hours
   d) 5 hours+

2. Do you think that becoming a celebrity—like a movie star or a rock star—would make you happier?
   a) Yes
   b) No
   c) I am not sure

3. If you could push a magic button that would change your life in one way, which of the following would you pick? *Please circle just one.*
   a) Becoming much smarter
   b) Becoming much bigger or stronger
   c) Becoming famous
   d) Becoming beautiful or more beautiful
   e) My life doesn't need any improving.

4. When you grow up, which of the following jobs would you MOST like to have? *Please circle just one.*
   a) The chief of a major company like General Motors
   b) The president of a great university like Harvard or Yale
   c) A Navy Seal
   d) A United States Senator
   e) The personal assistant to a very famous singer or movie star

5. Which of the following best describes your feelings about fame? *Please circle just one.*
   a) I don't really care about fame.
   b) I would like to become famous, but *only* if I *earned* it by becoming a good actor/actress or writing a best-selling book.
   c) I would like to become famous however I can, as long as I managed to get on TV.
   d) None of the above

6. When you watch TV comedies and dramas about kids your age, which reaction MOST represents how you feel?
   a) These kids are pretty cool and I wish they were my friends.
   b) In some ways, because I watch the show so much, I feel like they are my friends.
   c) Real life couldn't possibly be like this.
   d) None of the above

7. What are the odds that at some point in your life you will become famous? *Please circle just one.*
   a) It's very unlikely.
   b) I would say that I have a 25 percent chance.
   c) I would say that I have a 50 percent chance.
   d) I would say that I have a 75 percent chance.
   e) I'm not sure.

8. For those people who become celebrities, what BEST explains why? *Please circle just one.*
   a) They were simply lucky.
   b) They worked hard and they deserved it.
   c) They were born stars and it was just a matter of getting discovered.
   d) The entertainment industry simply decided to turn them into a star.
   e) I'm not sure.

9. On average, how often do you watch celebrity TV shows like *Entertainment Tonight, The Insider,* or *Access Hollywood*? *Please circle just one.*
    a) Never
    b) Once a month
    c) Once or twice a week
    d) Almost every day

10. On average, how often do you read magazines like *Us Weekly, Star, People, Teen People, YM,* or *J-14*?
    a) Never
    b) Once a month
    c) Once or twice a week
    d) Almost every day

11. When you watch TV shows or read magazine articles about the lives of celebrities, how do they make you feel? (Please write 1–3 sentences.)

12. How appreciated do you feel by your parents, friends, and teachers? *Please circle just one.*
    a) I feel VERY appreciated.
    b) I am basically appreciated enough.
    c) In truth, I am NOT appreciated enough.
    d) It seems like hardly anyone realizes my gifts or appreciates me.

13. How would you describe your family's situation with money?
    a) We don't have enough money.
    b) We have enough money.
    c) We have more than enough money.

14. At your school, how popular do you feel?
    a) Among the least popular
    b) Below average
    c) Average
    d) Above average
    e) Among the most popular
    f) I don't care to say.

15. At your school, how popular would you like to be?
    Please circle just one.
    a) It's not that important to me.
    b) I'd like to be averagely popular.
    c) I'd like to be among the most popular.
    d) In truth, I would like to be the most popular student in the whole school.
    e) I'm not sure or don't care.

16. If you became a celebrity, would kids at school like you more?
    a) Probably not
    b) Maybe
    c) Definitely
    d) Not sure

17. If you became a celebrity, would your family love you more?
    a) Probably not
    b) Maybe
    c) Definitely
    d) Not sure

18. How often do you get bullied or picked on by other kids?
    Please circle just one.
    a) Never
    b) Every once in a while
    c) Pretty often
    d) All the time

19. How many times have you gotten beaten up or really badly picked on? *Please circle just one.*
    a) 1–2 times
    b) 3–4 times
    c) 5–10 times
    d) More than 10 times
    e) I've never been beaten up.

20. If you suddenly became a celebrity—like a movie star or a rock star—what would be the best thing about being famous? (Please write 1–3 sentences.)

21. Do you have a favorite celebrity (singer, movie star, or sports star) whose career you follow or keep track of?
    a) Yes
    b) No
    c) I'm not sure.

22. Which of the following reasons BEST explains why you keep track of your favorite celebrity? *Please circle just one.*
    a) I just like watching this celebrity perform.
    b) I like to imagine myself hanging out with my favorite celebrity.
    c) My favorite celebrity just helps me feel good and forget about all of my troubles.
    d) I don't have a favorite celebrity.

23. If there were a way to have dinner with any of the following, who would you choose? *Please circle just one.*
    a) Jesus Christ
    b) Shaquille O'Neal
    c) 50 Cent
    d) Paris Hilton
    e) Albert Einstein
    f) Jennifer Lopez
    g) None
    h) President Bush

24. What kind of grades do you usually receive? *Please circle just one.*
    a) On average, I get mostly A's.
    b) On average, I get mostly B's.
    c) On average, I get mostly C's.
    d) On average, mostly D's.
    e) On average, mostly F's.

25. Which of the following imaginary people would you suspect is the most happy or content with their life?
    a) A man or woman who was just voted the best teacher at his school for the tenth year in a row
    b) A politician who just won the presidency of the United States
    c) A runner who just won a gold medal in the Olympics
    d) An actor or actress who just won an Oscar
    e) I am not sure.

26. Which of the following words sounds the most positive?
    a) Genius
    b) Celebrity
    c) Saint
    d) I am not sure.

27. Do you ever feel depressed, and if so, how often?
    a) I rarely or never feel depressed.
    b) I feel depressed sometimes.
    c) I feel depressed much of the time or pretty often.
    d) I almost always feel depressed.

28. Do you ever feel lonely, and if so, how often?
    a) I rarely or never feel lonely.
    b) I feel lonely sometimes.
    c) I feel lonely much of the time or pretty often.
    d) I almost always feel lonely.

29. Are you a boy or a girl?
    a) Boy
    b) Girl

30. How do you identify yourself ethnically or racially?
    a) Asian (includes Far East)
    b) Black/African-American
    c) Hispanic/Latino
    d) Native American
    e) White/Caucasian
    f) Mixed

31. What grade are you in?
    a) 5th
    b) 6th
    c) 7th
    d) 8th

32. To the best of your knowledge, what are the highest levels of your parents' (or caregivers') education? Please circle the highest level of education you believe they have completed.

Mother (or female caregiver)
    a) Some high school
    b) GED
    c) High school graduate
    d) Technical/trade school
    e) Some college
    f) Two-year degree
    g) Four-year degree
    h) Graduate school

Father (or male caregiver)
    a) Some high school
    b) GED
    c) High school graduate
    d) Technical/trade school
    e) Some college
    f) Two-year degree
    g) Four-year degree
    h) Graduate school

Thank you so much for your help!

Acknowledgments

I would like to start by thanking my editor, Heidi Pitlor, at Houghton Mifflin. She ushered this book through more drafts than I care to remember. At every step of the way she helped me make this a more thoughtful, intelligent, and well-written piece of work. She was tireless in her commitment to this book and, more important, to me as a writer. I feel very fortunate to have worked with her. I am also most grateful for the encouragement, advice, and unwavering friendship of two fellow writers—Elaine McArdle and Brian Groh—who read and reread these chapters with seemingly endless patience and enthusiasm. I can't emphasize enough how much that meant to me.

I would also like to give enormous thanks to my agent, Tina Bennett, who believed in this project from the beginning. She is simply the smartest, shrewdest, and most supportive advocate any person could hope to have. Writing is by its very nature a lonely endeavor, and I always took great comfort knowing that Tina was with me at every step along the way. Her assistant, Svetlana Katz, is also an insightful reader whose help I much appreciated.

I would like to thank several magazine and radio editors for their time and thoughts: Sara Sarasohn, of National Public Radio, who helped me find my voice and my confidence in writing about Hollywood; Dana Goodyear, of *The New Yorker;* Jon Marcus, of *Boston Magazine;* Diana Delling, of *Outside Magazine;* and Vera Titunik, of the *New York Times Magazine.* I am also indebted to my friend and mentor, Joseph Finder, who helped me think through virtually every problem I encountered.

While writing this book I was often on the road, which can be immensely tiring, and a few friends provided me with true homes away from home. Charles and Tara Wachter took me in like family, and put me up for weeks at a time in Los Angeles. Their generosity was astounding. During my time in the Southwest, Stephen and Stephanie Glass allowed me to stay in their guesthouse in Cortez, Colorado. No one could wish for a more peaceful place to work. And I will never forget Micah Nathan and Rachel Kane, for sharing their cozy apartment in Boston on many a wintry evening. Those nights sustained me.

In the research for this book I was aided immensely by a number of academics. Robert Thompson, of Syracuse University, was a great help. Somehow, he always found time to answer my calls and offer thoughtful advice. Jean Twenge, of San Diego State University, was endlessly helpful with her research on narcissism and self-esteem. I would also like to thank Tom Sander, of Harvard University; Francisco Gil-White, of the University of Pennsylvania; Robert Millman, of Cornell; Hans Breiter and Daphne Holt, of Massachusetts General Hospital; Daniel Lapsley, of Ball State University; Keith Campbell, of the University of Georgia; Stephen Kent, of the University of Alberta; Robert Cialdini and Douglas Kenrick, of Arizona State University; Michael Platt, of Duke; and Lynn McCutcheon, of the DeVry Institute of Technology, in Orlando.

I could not have conducted my survey in Rochester, New York, without the help of Elaine Allen, of Babson College. She helped me analyze the data, understand the implications, and couch my arguments. Andrew MacGowan; Linda McKenzie; Janine Sanger; Meredith Hight; Carol Liebler, of Syracuse University; Carlos Brain and Nirupama Rao, of MIT; and Richard McGowan, of Boston College, were also of help with the survey.

While I was in the field, conducting interviews, a number of people shared their stories and insights. I am indebted to all of them. In particular I would like to thank Cal Merlander, Susan

Makai, Russell Turiak, Marcy Braunstein, David Jones, Michael Levine, the Edge, Dean Johnson, Ed Zwick, Annie Brentwell, and Bill Gordon. I am also grateful to Emmett McAuliffe for his observations on fame and the music business.

A few key people made a big difference in the actual publishing of this book. I'd like to thank Megan Wilson, publicist extraordinaire, whose energy, creativity, and friendship have always meant a great deal to me. My new editor, Webster Younce, helped me apply the finishing touches on this book. I so appreciate all of his help and I look forward to working with him in the future. Martha Spaulding did a meticulous job copyediting my manuscript. Nicole Angeloro went out of her way to help me on many occasions and provided the kind of smart, excellent support I have come to expect at Houghton Mifflin. And once again Carla Gray worked wonders on the marketing front.

Finally, I would like to thank my family. Tammy Halpern and Paul Zuydhoek did more for me than they realize, by building our idyllic family home in Great Barrington and always keeping its doors open. That place is my refuge from the world. Stephen Halpern and Betty Stanton have steadily been there for me — listening to my writing, offering encouragement, and whisking me off to Norbie's. Barbara Lipska, Mirek Gorski, and Witek Lipski always respected and believed in my work. Thank you for that. My brother, to whom this book is dedicated, is a friend and a shining example of artistic integrity. And last I'd like to thank my wife, Kasia Lipska, whose love, adventuresome spirit, and quirky Polish witticisms got me through all the days when it wasn't looking good.

Notes

Introduction: Hooked on Fame

xv *American Idol:* This statistic was derived by comparing the average viewership of *American Idol* finales from 2002 to 2005 with the average viewership of NBC's *Nightly News,* ABC's *World News Tonight,* and CBS's *Evening News* for the third and fourth quarters of 2005. The viewership of the *American Idol* finales was as follows: (2002) Justin Guarini vs. Kelly Clarkson: 22.8 million. Source: "Big 'Idol' Winner: Fox Talent-show Finale Hit Ratings High," *New York Daily News,* September 6, 2002. (2003) Ruben Studdard vs. Clay Aiken: 38.1 million. Source: "Stunning Success of 'American Idol' Gives Fox an Easy Ratings Win," Associated Press, May 28, 2003. (2004) Fantasia Barrino vs. Diana DeGarmo: 31.4 million. Source: "'Idol' Season Chart-Topper," *The Hollywood Reporter,* May 28, 2004. (2005) Carrie Underwood vs. Bo Bice: 30.3 million. Source: "Viewers Flock to Network TV for Finale of Television Season," Associated Press, June 1, 2005. The average of these four finales was 30.65 million. The viewership of the major news shows was as follows:

	NBC Nightly News	ABC World News Tonight	CBS Evening News	TOTAL
3rd Quarter '05	8.6 million	8.1 million	6.6 million	23.3 million
4th Quarter '05	9.79 million	8.65 million	7.47 million	25.91 million

Compiled using information from Michele Greppi, "'NBC Nightly News' Big 3's Most Seen," *Television Week,* October 3, 2005 (3rd quarter) and "'Nightly News' Tops in Q4 Ratings Battle," *Television Week,* January 2, 2006 (4th quarter).

xv the circulation of the major entertainment: This information was obtained courtesy of Ruth McFarland, of Bacon's Information.

Publication	2000 Circulation	2005 Circulation
News		
The New Yorker	813,044	1,054,167
Atlantic Monthly	463,587	405,723

Publication	2000 Circulation	2005 Circulation
Newsweek	3,178,207	3,200,413
Time	4,083,387	4,050,589
TOTAL	8,538,225	8,710,892
Entertainment		
InStyle	1,360,163	1,793,002
People	3,659,151	3,779,640
Us Weekly	1,100,000	1,662,003
Entertainment Weekly	1,532,835	1,852,376
TOTAL	7,652,149	9,087,021

xv celebrity labels: Stephanie Thompson, "Who Are You Wearing? Why, It's a Gwen," *Advertising Age,* September 12, 2005.

xv Gallup Organization: Data was provided by The Roper Center for Public Opinion Research, at the University of Connecticut. It is based on a poll conducted by the Gallup Organization. The poll asked, "What man that you have heard or read about, living today in any part of the world, do you admire most?" The most recent poll was conducted December 19 through December 22, 2005, through telephone interviews with a national adult sample of 1,004 people. The earlier poll was conducted December 5 through December 10, 1963, through personal interviews with a national adult sample of 1,613 people.

xviii the Hadza tribe: For more information on the Hadza see Susan Kent, *Ethnicity, Hunter-Gatherers, and the "Other": Association or Assimilation in Africa* (Washington, D.C.: Smithsonian Institution Press, 2002), 247–275.

xx *Photoplay:* I obtained back issues of *Photoplay* courtesy of the library at Bowling Green University. The circulation of *People* comes from *Bacon's Magazine Directory.*

xx emergence of cable television: Sally Bedell Smith, "Reporter's Notebook: Cable Meeting," *New York Times,* June 18, 1983; Bob Keefe, "Niche Channels Face Large Odds," *The Atlanta Journal-Constitution,* April 2, 2005.

xx In the early 1970s: Gail Pennington, "TV Guide Tunes in to the 21st Century: With the Proliferation of Cable Channels, the Magazine Is Reducing its Listings and Adding More Features," *St. Louis Post-Dispatch,* October 9, 2005.

xxi U.S. Department of Labor: This report can be found at www.bls.gov/oco/cg/cgs038.htm#outlook.

xxi Screen Actors Guild: Jesse Hiestand, "Reality Still Biting SAG," *Hollywood Reporter,* October 6, 2005; "Actors Face Reality," *New York Times,* October 7, 2005.

xxi September 11, 2001: Jim Greenman, *What Happened to the World?: Helping Children Cope in Turbulent Times* (Watertown, Mass.: Bright Horizons Family Solutions, 2001). www.brighthorizons.com/talktochildren/docs/whathapp.pdf.

xxii *Journal of the American Medical Association:* Scott Stossel, "The Man Who Counts the Killings," *Atlantic Monthly,* May 1997.

xxv "giant pharmaceutical factory": Harvey Milkman and Stanley Sunderwirth, *Craving for Ecstasy: How Our Passions Become Addictions and What We Can Do About Them* (San Francisco: Jossey-Bass, 1998), xiii.

xxv *Addictive Personality:* Craig Nakken, *Addictive Personality: Understanding the Addictive Process and Compulsive Behavior* (Center City, Minn.: Hazelden, 1996).

xxvii Many health care experts: On its Web site the National Institutes of Health notes that there is "substantial evidence that reducing alcohol availability can reduce alcohol consumption." grants.nih.gov/grants/guide/pa-files/PA-05-146.html.

xxvii "The more available addictive": Nakken, *Addictive Personality.*

xxviii "thousands of fame-wheels": *The Poet's Guide to Life: The Wisdom of Rilke by Rainer Maria Rilke,* trans. Ulrich Baer (New York: Modern Library, 2005).

PART I: THE WORLD OF ASPIRING
CHILD CELEBRITIES

1: Going to Fame School

4 Representatives from Barbizon: Karin Chenoweth, "Not a Good Model for Use of School Time," *Washington Post,* May 22, 2003.

5 In his 1960 classic: John Robert Powers, *How to Have Model Beauty, Poise, & Personality: Tested Methods the Models Use by the World's Most Famous Expert on Feminine Appearance* (Englewood Cliffs, N.J.: Prentice-Hall, 1960).

15 Both theories first appeared: David Elkind, "Egocentrism in Adolescence," *Child Development,* 38, no. 4 (1967): 1025–1034.

16 To test these theories: Lesa Rae Vartanian, "Revisiting the Imaginary Audience and Personal Fable Constructs of Adolescent Egocentrism: A Conceptual Review," *Adolescence,* 35, no. 140 (Winter 2000): 639–661.

18 Sadly, studies show: T. Riley, G. R. Adams, and E. Nielsen, "Adolescent Egocentrism: The Association Among Imaginary Audience Behavior, Cognitive Development, and Parental Support and Rejection," *Journal of Youth and Adolescence,* 13 (October 1984): 401–417.

18 "special vulnerability": Laurence Steinberg et al., *The Study of Developmental Psychopathology in Adolescence: Integrating Affective Neuroscience with the Study of Context* (New York: John Wiley & Sons, 2004).

2: Mobs of Fame-Starved Children

34 Marilyn Monroe: As quoted in Gloria Steinem, "The Woman Who Will Not Die," in *All the Available Light: A Marilyn Monroe Reader,* ed. Yona Zeldis McDonough (New York: Touchstone, 2002), 63.

34 celebrities who claim to have overcome: For more information on the hard childhoods of the named celebrities, see: (Gregory Peck) Sterlin Holmesly, "Peck Bio a Sloppy Mess," *San Antonio (Texas) Express-News,* December 19, 2004; (Audrey Hepburn) Liz Braun, "Our Liz Recommends . . . ," *Toronto Sun,* December 21, 2003; (Billie Holiday) Allis Moss, "East Coast Blues," *The Independent* (London), May 27, 2000; (Mariah Carey) Rebecca Louie, "Mariah Wins Her Wings," *(New York) Daily News,* April 10, 2005; (Halle Berry) "The People Beat," *San Antonio (Texas) Express-News,* February 12, 2002; (Roman Polanski) Jay Boyar, "Polanski's Work Reflects a Life of Triumphs and Tragedies," *Pittsburgh Post-Gazette,* April 20, 2003; (Sean Combs) "Bad Boy Worldwide Entertainment Group," *Time,* December 20, 2004; (Jim Carrey) Jamie Portman, "Carrey's Almighty Passion: Canadian Superstar Reveals the Day His Prayers Come True," *Ottawa Citizen,* May 21, 2003.

35 Minnesota Multiphasic Personality Inventory: Cassandra Rutledge Newsom et al., "Changes in Adolescent Response Patterns on the MMPI/MMPI-A Across Four Decades," *Journal of Personality,* 81 (August 2003): 74–84.

35 Twenge speculated: Jean Twenge and Keith Campbell, "Age and Birth Cohort Differences in Self-esteem: A Cross-temporal Meta-analysis," *Personality and Social Psychology Review,* 5 (November 2001): 321–44.

36 *Generation Me:* Jean Twenge, *Generation Me: Why Today's Young Americans Are More Confident, Assertive, Entitled—and More Miserable Than Ever Before* (New York: Free Press, 2006).

37 *American Educator:* Lilian Katz, "All About Me: Are We Developing our Children's Self-esteem or Their Narcissism?" *American Educator,* 17, no. 2 (1993): 18–23.

37 Harrison Gough: As quoted in Twenge, *Generation Me.*

37 Narcissism Personality Inventory: Joshua D. Foster, W. Keith Campbell, and Jean M. Twenge, "Individual Differences in Narcissism: Inflated Self-views Across the Lifespan and Around the World," *Journal of Research in Personality,* 37 (2003): 469–86.

38 "to maintain a constant flow": Katz, "All About Me."

39 Eysenck Personality Questionnaire: Jean Twenge, "Birth Cohort Changes in Extraversion: A Cross-temporal meta-analysis, 1966–1993," *Personality and Individual Differences,* 30 (2001): 735–48.

39 *Loveline* celebrities: S. Mark Young and Drew Pinsky, "Narcissism and Celebrity." Currently under review at the *Journal of Research in Personality.*

42 "The people who run": C. I. Walker and Natasha Esch, *The Wilhelmina Guide to Modeling* (New York: Fireside, 1996).

3: A Home for the Famous and the Almost Famous

72 Craig Nakken makes: Craig Nakken, *Addictive Personality: Understanding the Addictive Process and Compulsive Behavior* (Center City, Minn.: Hazelden, 1996).

73 Sally Field: Sharon Waxman, "The Lost Art of Saying Thank You; The Oscar Acceptance Speech: Off and Running at the Mouth," *Washington Post*, March 21, 1999.

PART II: THE CELEBRITY ENTOURAGE

4: The Association of Celebrity Personal Assistants

81 In Roman times: Christopher Buckley, "My Entourage Is Bigger Than Your Entourage," *Business Review Weekly*, November 16, 1998.

87 Despite all the bad behavior: R. Dean Johnson, *Life. Be There at Ten 'Til: A Collection of Homegrown Wisdom* (Lincoln, Neb.: iUniverse Star, 2005).

98 Stephen Kent studies: Stephen Kent, "Scientology—Is This a Religion?" *Marburg Journal of Religion*, 4 (July 1999).

5: The Desire to Belong: Why Everyone Wants to Have Dinner with Paris Hilton and 50 Cent

112 Belongingness Theory: Roy F. Baumeister and Mark R. Leary, "The Need to Belong: Desire for Interpersonal Attachments as a Fundamental Human Motivation," *Psychological Bulletin* 117 (May 1995): 497–529.

113 "social affect and": Jaak Panksepp, "Brain Opioids and Social Emotions," as cited in *The Psychobiology of Attachment and Separation*, ed. M. Reite and T. Field, 3–49 (New York: Academic Press, 1985).

113 "The persona offers": Donald Horton and R. Richard Wohl, "Mass Communication and Para-social Interaction: Observations on Intimacy at a Distance," *Psychiatry* 19 (1956): 215–29.

114 Soap-opera viewers: David Giles, *Illusions of Immortality: A Psychology of Fame and Celebrity* (New York: St. Martin's Press, 2000), 64.

115 Another major change: Robert E. Lane, *The Loss of Happiness in Market Democracies* (New Haven, Conn.: Yale University Press, 2000), 85.

115 In 1956 the median age: Information courtesy of Cheryl Russell, Editorial Director, New Strategist Publications, www.newstrategist.com. For additional information on the demographics of young Americans today see: New Strategist Editors, *Generation X: Americans Born 1965 to 1976*, 4th ed. (Ithaca, N.Y.: New Strategist Publications, 2004), 172.

115 The share of American households: Philip Cushman, "Why the Self Is Empty: Toward a Historically Situated Psychology," *American Psychologist* 45

(1990): 599; U.S. Census Bureau, "HH-4: Households by Size: 1960 to Present."
www.census.gov/population/socdemo/hh-fam/hh4.pdf.

115 Since 1970 the number of youths:

	1970 People Living Alone	2005 People Living Alone
Ages 15–24	556,000 (1.4 percent of age group)	1,502,000 (3.7 percent of age group)
Ages 25–34	893,000 (3.6 percent of age group)	3,772,000 (9.6 percent of age group)

Compiled using information courtesy of Cheryl Russell, New Strategist Publications.

115 The combination of loneliness: D. D. Ashe and Lynn McCutcheon, "Shyness, Loneliness, and Attitude Toward Celebrities," *Current Research in Social Psychology* 6, no. 9 (2001). Note: The correlation that McCutcheon and Ashe found was significant, but not overwhelmingly strong.

116 "Perhaps one of the ways": Lynn McCutcheon et al., "Preference for Solitude and Attitude Toward One's Favorite Celebrity," *North American Journal of Psychology* 6, no. 3 (2004): 499–505.

116 Another investigation: Jacki Fitzpatrick and Andrea McCourt, "The Role of Personal Characteristics and Romantic Characteristics in Parasocial Relationships: A Pilot Study," *Journal of Mundane Behavior* 2 (February 2001).

120 One could argue: Pamela Bettis and Natalie Adams, "The Power of the Preps and a Cheerleading Equity Policy," *Sociology of Education* 76 (April 2003): 128–142.

120 In a landmark study: Donna Eder, "The Cycle of Popularity: Interpersonal Relations Among Female Adolescents," *Sociology of Education* 58 (July 1985): 152–65.

121 Prestige Theory: J. Henrich and F. J. Gil-White, "The Evolution of Prestige: Freely Conferred Status as a Mechanism for Enhancing the Benefits of Cultural Transmission," *Evolution and Human Behavior* 22, no. 3 (2001): 165–96.

122 an experiment conducted by two Emory primatologists: Josep Call and Michael Tomasello, "Use of Social Information in the Problem Solving of Orangutans (*Pongo pygmaeus*) and Human Children (Homo sapiens)," *Journal of Comparative Psychology* 109 (September 1995): 308–20.

6: When Reflected Glory Isn't Enough: Confessions of an Upwardly Mobile Celebrity "Slave"

126 In the mid-1970s Cialdini: Robert B. Cialdini and Richard J. Borden, "Basking in Reflected Glory: Three (Football) Field Studies," *Journal of Personality and Social Psychology* 34, no. 3 (1976): 366–75.

126 Cialdini soon began: Cialdini and Borden, "Basking in Reflected Glory."

127 Douglas Schofield: Robert B. Cialdini and Maralou E. De Nicholas, "Self-Presentation by Association," *Journal of Personality and Social Psychology* 57, no. 4 (1989): 626–31.

128 Grigori Rasputin: John F. Finch and Robert B. Cialdini, "Another Indirect Tactic of (Self-) Image Management: Boosting," *Personality and Social Psychology Bulletin* 15 (June 1989): 222–32.

PART III: THE WORLD OF CELEBRITY WORSHIPERS

7: Monkeys, *Us Weekly,* and the Power of Social Information

141 When it comes to knowing: William A. Gordon, *The Ultimate Hollywood Tour Book* (Lake Forrest, Calif.: North Ridge Books, 2002).

144 According to the search engine: This information comes from Yahoo!'s "Buzz Index," which publishes a list of top search terms for each year. The list for 2005 is available at tools.search.yahoo.com/top2005/.

144 In his book Putnam: Information on the DDB life-style study was obtained through the generous help of Thomas Sander, of the John F. Kennedy School of Government at Harvard University, and DDB, in Chicago.

145 There is evidence that: Jean Twenge, Kathleen Catanese, and Roy Baumeister, "Social Exclusion Causes Self-defeating Behavior," *Journal of Personality and Social Psychology* 83 (September 2002): 606–15. Note: Additional information came from extensive interviews with Jean Twenge.

145 Twenge's interest in celebrities: Jean Twenge et al., "Replenishing Connectedness: Reminders of Social Activity Reduce Aggression After Social Exclusion," *British Journal of Social Psychology.* In press.

147 The psychologist Robin Dunbar: Robin Dunbar, "Gossip in Evolutionary Perspective," *Review of General Psychology* 8 (June 2004): 100–110.

148 During the first six months of 2005: Roben Farzad, "To Market a Magazine, Fill It With Celebrity Gossip," *New York Times,* August 16, 2005; Ruth McFarland, at Bacon's Information.

150 In the very early days: Joshua Gamson, *Claims to Fame: Celebrity in Contemporary America* (Berkeley, Calif.: University of California Press, 1994), 24.

150 Sometime around 1909: Richard deCordova, *Picture Personalities: The Emergence of the Star System in America* (Urbana, Ill.: University of Illinois Press, 2001).

150 "Loretta Young is": "The Beauty Who Cannot Stay in Love," *Photoplay,* September 1935. Note: I obtained a copy of this magazine courtesy of the library at Bowling Green University.

150 In 1940 *Life*: Gamson, *Claims to Fame,* 29.

151 "Liz Will Adopt a Negro Baby!": *Movie Mirror,* April 1967. "Why Shirley Jones's Sex Opinions Broke Up Her Marriage," *Movie Life,* May 1972. "Cops Seize Onassis's Dirty Picture Collection," *Motion Picture,* February 1971.

153 In 2005 he and his: R. O. Deaner, A. V. Khera, and M. L. Platt, "Monkeys Pay per View: Adaptive Valuation of Social Images by Rhesus Macaques," *Current Biology* 15 (March 29, 2005): 543–48.

156 Another explanation is: Jeannie Williams, "The Scoop on the 'Gladiator' Dog," *USA Today,* May 10, 2000 (Tom Cruise); Trish Donnally, "The Award for Best Oscar Gowns Goes to . . . VERA WANG," *San Francisco Chronicle,* April 11, 2000 (Sharon Stone); Sharon Fink, "Oscar Night Approaches," *St. Petersburg (Florida) Times,* February 24, 2005 (gift baskets); "Hold the Phone: Crowe Also Threw a Vase," *Daily Telegraph* (Sydney, Australia), June 30, 2005 (Russell Crowe).

156 the demeanor of some: Frans de Waal, *Chimpanzee Politics: Power and Sex among Apes* (Baltimore, Md.: Johns Hopkins University Press, 2000): 47.

8: A Choice of Worship: Rod *vs.* God

164 Prominence of evangelical Christianity: All data come from the online archives of the Gallup Organization. Three different polling questions were described: (1) "How important would you say religion is in your own life—very important, fairly important, or not very important?" In 1952 this question was polled repeatedly, and on average 75 percent said religion was very important. In 2005, between May 2 and 5, 55 percent said religion was very important. (2) "At the present time, do you think religion as a whole is increasing its influence on American life or losing its influence?" In 1957, between March 15 and 20, 14 percent of subjects indicated that religion was losing its influence. In 2005, between April 18 and 21, 46 percent said religion was losing its influence. (3) "Do you believe that religion can answer all or most of today's problems, or that religion is largely old-fashioned and out of date?" In 1957, between March 15 and 20, 82 percent said that religion "can answer" today's problems and 7 percent said it was "out of date." In 2005, between April 18 and 21, 58 percent said that religion "can answer" today's problems and 23 percent said it was "out of date."

165 In the mid-1990s Jindra: M. Jindra, "*Star Trek* Fandom as a Religious Phenomenon," *Sociology of Religion* 55 (Spring 1994): 27.

166 In 2001 John Maltby: John Maltby et al., "Thou Shalt Worship No Other Gods—Unless They Are Celebrities: The Relationship Between Celebrity Worship and Religious Orientation," *Personality and Individual Differences* 32 (May 2002): 1157–72.

166 The questions about religion: Richard Beck and Ryan Jessup, "The Multidimensional Nature of Quest Motivation," *Journal of Psychology & Theology* 32 (Winter 2004): 283–94.

178 "Fan," which first came: Laura Leets et al., "Fans: Exploring Expressed Motivations for Contacting Celebrities," *Journal of Language and Social Psychology* 14 (March 1995): 102–23.

178 In California, at least: California Penal Code § 646.9. Stalking. 1990. Amended 2002.

178 Some experts surmise: Kerry O. Ferris, "Through a Glass, Darkly: The Dynamics of Fan-Celebrity Encounters," *Symbolic Interaction* 24, no. 1 (2001): 25–47.

181 Kris Mohandie has made a name: K. Mohandie et al., "The RECON Typology of Stalking: Reliability and Validity Based Upon a Large Sample of North American Stalkers," *Journal of Forensic Sciences* 51 (2006): 147–55.

Conclusion: Some Reflections from Hollywood's Premier Retirement Home

187 "Now you will not swell": A. E. Housman, *A Shropshire Lad* (New York: Buccaneer Books, 1983).

188 *Us Weekly*'s coverage: For more information on how *Us Weekly* covered the 2005 MTV Video Music Awards see: Ariana Eunjung Cha, "Print Media's Hot New Star: Celebrity Mags; Glossies Like Us Weekly Gaining Circulation," *Washington Post,* September 23, 2005.

188 Nielsen Media Research found: This information was provided courtesy of Alex Still, at Nielsen Media.

188 NBA finals: Gary Levin, "NBA Sizzles; Bride Fizzles," *USA Today,* June 29, 2005. Miss America Pageant: "'Idol,' NFL Make Fox No. 1," *Los Angeles Times,* January 25, 2006. Ken Burns's series on jazz: "'Jazz' Doubles PBS Audience," *San Diego Union-Tribune,* January 18, 2001.

193 January 7, 2005: On *CNN Saturday Morning News* hosts Tony Harris and Betty Nguyen and CNN correspondent Brooke Anderson discussed Brad Pitt and Jennifer Aniston's breakup. Their actual dialogue, excluding prompts like "begin videotape," was 419 words long. CNN's transcripts reveal that the network devoted just sixty-one words to the Max Baucus story (*Judy Woodruff's Inside Politics,* CNN, January 7, 2005), sixty-five words to the Katrina Leung story (*American Morning,* CNN, January 7, 2005), and just fifty-five words to the oil-for-food story (*CNN Capital Gang,* January 8, 2005, devoted twenty-four words; *CNN Live Saturday,* January 8, 2005, devoted thirty-one words). On those two days there was no mention in CNN's transcripts of the AIDS research story or the federal pension-insurance program story.

193 the *New York Times:* "News Summary," *New York Times,* January 7, 2005: A2.

193 Greta Van Susteren: *On the Record with Greta Van Susteren,* Fox, January 7, 2005 (10:51 P.M. EST).

194 The following day CNN's: *CNN Saturday Morning News,* January 8, 2005 (7:00 A.M. EST).

194 Andrew Tyndall: The stats about Darfur were cited most prominently in Nicholas D. Kristoff, "All Ears for Tom Cruise, All Eyes on Brad Pitt," *New York Times,* July 26, 2005. Additional information courtesy of Andrew Tyndall.

Top Ten News Stories of 2004	Total Minutes	Good Morning America (ABC)	The Early Show (CBS)	The Today Show (NBC)
1 Election Campaign of 2004	3015	924	694	1398
2 War in Iraq: the post-war insurgency, terrorism, and reconstruction	1103	380	280	442
3 The Athens Summer Olympic Games	869	49	77	743
4 The Laci Peterson Murder Case	845	245	303	297
5 Michael Jackson Child Molestation Trial	563	205	146	213
6 Martha Stewart Trial	481	180	124	176
7 The 9/11 Commission Report	464	159	113	192
8 Former President Ronald Reagan's Death	359	149	109	101
9 Recipes and Cooking Tips	339	91	178	70
10 Abu Ghraib Story	336	114	66	156

Source: Andrew Tyndall

196 The *New York Times* noted: Bill Carter, "Why Hold the Superlatives? 'American Idol' Is Ascendant," *New York Times,* January 30, 2006.

196 According to a Washington Post: "Survey of Teens in the Greater Washington, D.C., Area," Washington Post/Kaiser Family Foundation/Harvard University Survey, October 2005. This is available online, www.kff.org/kaiser-polls/upload/-Survey-of-Teens-in-the-Greater-Washington-DC-Area-Toplines.pdf. In answer to the question: "How likely is it that you will be famous someday? Is it very likely, fairly likely, not too likely, or not likely at all?" 31 percent said "very likely" or "likely."

197 Keith Campbell: Joshua D. Foster, W. Keith Campbell, and Jean M. Twenge, "Individual Differences in Narcissism: Inflated Self-views Across the Lifespan and Around the World," *Journal of Research in Personality* 37 (2003): 469–86.

197 "We are the middle children": Chuck Palahniuk, *Fight Club* (New York: Owl Books, 2004), 157.